Gestational Diabetes explained.

Gestational Diabetes symptoms, diet, meal plan, causes, diagnosis, treatments, managing GD, medication and emotional health all included.

by

Robert Rymore

Acknowledgements

Thanks to my wife and children for supporting me.

Thanks to Haider, my co-writer, for his extensive knowledge on Gestational Diabetes.

Table of Contents

Table of Contents

Table of Contents

Table of Contents

Table of Contents

Table of Contents

Chapter 1: Introduction

Much has been written about pregnancy and its complications, risk factors, general health guidelines, nutritional aspects and whatnot. However, you will very rarely find a comprehensive account of a pregnancy-related medical condition that is free of technical jargon, complicated statistics and confusing recommendations. Gestational Diabetes is a condition that has been on the rise, like other types of diabetes, for the last few decades and poses a significant threat to both mother and the fetus. There is high demand for a good quality book that covers all the related information on its different aspects without being very technical or complicated. There is more than enough medical literature on gestational diabetes but for a common housewife planning to get pregnant, there are very few reliable sources available that can be trusted. This book is a comprehensive guide, covering information on Gestational Diabetes, controlling and managing all possible risk factors and proper assistance regarding dietary recommendations. For those mothers who don't have this disease, it allow them to seek protection from gestational diabetes when they go through one of the most important periods of their lives. For those who, unfortunately, suffer from this disease, it provides a clear path that can safely bring them to their destination. This book plans to help you in managing your Gestational diabetes and at the same time you can gain enjoyable health for you and your child.

1) A brief description regarding the importance of a healthy pregnancy

International statistics reveal that every year over ***one hundred and thirty million*** births take place all over the world. Statistics for the United States are nearly *four million* births annually. An alarming ratio among these births is complicated by several medical disorders. Most of these medical conditions and disorders were contraindicated to pregnancy in the past. Countless clinical studies and advances in medicine, obstetric anesthesiology, obstetrics and neonatology have led to higher expectations that a successful pregnancy can bring a positive outcome for both child and the mother, despite underlying medical disorders. There are several medical complications that can negatively impact the physiological adaptations of pregnancy, and that can adversely affect an underlying medical condition. The most common of such medical disorders are:

Hypertension, Chronic Essential hypertension

Preeclampsia, Gestational Hypertension

Renal Disease, Cardiac Disease (Congenital Heart Disease, Valvular Heart Disease, Mitral Stenosis, Mitral regurgitation and Aortic regurgitation and Stenosis, Other Cardiac Disorders)

Specific High risk Cardiac Lesions, Marfan syndrome

Pulmonary Hypertension

Pulmonary Embolism and Deep Venous Thrombosis

Endocrine Disorders (Diabetes Mellitus in Pregnancy)

Gestational Diabetes

Hyperthyroidism in Pregnancy (thyroid disease)

Obesity, Neurological Disorders

Hematologic Disorders, Infections (Bacterial infections, Viral Infections)

Viral Infections including *Cytomegalovirus infection, Rubella, Herpes virus, Parvo virus, HIV AIDS*

Liver and Gastrointestinal Diseases.

a) Hypertension

During pregnancy, the heartrate increases by ten beats per minute and cardiac output is elevated by forty percent (40%) in the 3rd trimester. This is due to an increase in stroke volume.

Definition of STROKE VOLUME: "The volume of blood pumped from a ventricle of the heart in one beat."

Systemic vascular resistance drops due to a decrease in blood pressure during the 2nd trimester. For a pregnant female, blood pressure of 140/90 mmHg is considered alarming, which is linked to an increase in perinatal morbidity and mortality.

b) Preeclampsia

The proportion of preeclampsia in pregnant women is around 5 to 7 percent. Preeclampsia is an initial stage of proteinuria and hypertension, following 20 weeks of gestation.

Definition of PREECLAMPSIA: "A serious condition developing in late pregnancy that is characterized by a sudden rise in blood pressure, excessive weight gain, generalized edema, proteinuria, severe headaches and visual disturbances and that may result in eclampsia (a : convulsions or coma late in pregnancy in an individual affected by preeclampsia) if untreated"—

c) Renal disease

Almost 3% of pregnancies are complicated by hypertension resulting in maternal, fetal and neonatal deaths. Pregnant mothers suffering from underlying hypertension and renal disease may experience worsening of their hypertension.

d) Cardiac Disease

Mitral Stenosis is among those cardiac (Valvular) diseases that can result in death during pregnancy. Sudden deaths have taken place in the past and the reason is that during pregnancy, the volume of blood increases and so does the cardiac output.

e) Marfan syndrome

During pregnancy almost 15 percent of females with underlying *Marfan syndrome* can undergo serious cardiovascular manifestations.

Definition of MARFAN SYNDROME: "A disorder of connective tissue that is inherited as a simple dominant trait, is caused by a defect in the gene controlling the production of fibrillin, and is characterized by abnormal elongation of the long bones and often by ocular and circulatory defects."

f) The Endocrine Disorders (diabetes mellitus)

Most of the complications in pregnancy that are caused by diabetes mellitus are associated with perinatal morbidity. Gestational diabetes causes significant healthcare problems throughout the world and needs to be tackled effectively.

g) Obesity:

Obese pregnant females are at a greater risk of post-date delivery, urinary tract infections, gestational diabetes and congenital fetal malformations. All of these complications are harmful for both mother and fetus.

2) Definitions

"Gestational diabetes is a type of diabetes that affects women during pregnancy. Diabetes is a condition where there is too much glucose (sugar) in the blood.

Normally, the amount of glucose in the blood is controlled by a hormone called insulin. However, during pregnancy, some women have higher than normal levels of glucose in their blood and their body cannot produce enough insulin to transport it all into the cells. This means that the level of glucose in the blood rises". *Source: www.nhs.co.uk*

Explanations of the various definitions of gestational diabetes in medical literature:

According to Harrison's Principles of Internal Medicine, "*Insulin resistance is related to the metabolic changes of late pregnancy and the increased insulin requirements may lead to IGT. Gestational diabetes mellitus (GDM) occurs in 4% of pregnancies in the United States; most women revert to normal glucose tolerance post-partum but have a substantial risk (30–60%) of developing DM later in life*". The percentage of Gestation Diabetes in pregnant women is continuously increasing at an alarming rate. An estimated 17,000 females developed Gestational Diabetes in Australia last year alone. Gestational Diabetes can be related to several high risk complications in pregnant mothers and their children. Unfortunately, the child has a greater threat of developing diabetes at a later stage in his/her life. A comprehensive treatment and management plan is required to noticeably reduce and avoid such health hazards for the newborn. Huge advancements have been made recently in the field of Gestational Diabetes management. Influential knowledge has been gained through clinical studies explaining different treatment options, highlighting the significance of a healthy lifestyle and establishing pros and cons of eating habits.

3) Latest Statistics

Latest statistics highlighting prevalence, morbidity, mortality and effects on final pregnancy outcomes: Statistics gathered by *World Health Organization* in 1997 about the prevalence of diabetes revealed an estimated increase of more than 120% from one hundred and thirty five million in 1995 to nearly three hundred million by the year 2025. These horrifying statistics include GD statistics as well. Therefore, now there is a special need of direct and significant attention to be paid to this portion of population, especially to reduce possible, fatal outcomes.

* UNITED STATES: Prevalence rate of Gestational Diabetes:

In the United States, 2 to 10 % of pregnant women have been reported to suffer from gestational diabetes in 2011.

There is a 35-60 % chance of developing diabetes in females who have had gestational diabetes at some point in their lives. Diabetes in such females can take place within 10-20 years of their gestational diabetes.

Research studies under new international diagnostic criteria have reported that currently more than 18% of pregnancies are affected by gestational diabetes.

4) An overview of what's new in the gestational diabetes phenomena

The most disturbing fact about GD is that it is on the rise. In 1985 there were about 30 million cases of GD worldwide and the number jumped to 177 million in 2000. At this rate, 360 million mothers will suffer from GD by the start of 2030. According to the National Center for Chronic Disease Prevention and Health Promotion's Diabetes Report Card 2012, *"Gestational diabetes develops and is diagnosed as a result of pregnancy in 2%–10% of pregnant women in US"*. This is a significant increase compared to rest of the world, where the latest data is not yet available. A universal trend of increasing diabetes cases has been observed in its subtypes as well, including GD. Out of 25.6 million Americans suffering from diabetes in 2010, 12.6 million were women.

This book has been written to guide you to take important precautionary measures to prevent complications caused by gestational diabetes. I hope that you'll find the contents extremely beneficial for both yourself and your soon to be born baby.

Chapter 2: Pregnancy And Its Complications

1) Pregnancy

Pregnancy is the process of the fertilization and development of an embryo in woman's uterus. "Gestation" is another term used for pregnancy. Pregnancy lasts for about 40 weeks and it starts from the first day of your last normal period and is grouped into **three trimesters**.

The *first trimester*- the first few months of pregnancy- involves rapid physical changes in your body inducing nausea, fatigue and rapid mood swings. The first trimester is the time of rapid development and growth for your baby as the baby's spinal cord, brain and other organs begin to form. Your baby's heart begins to beat and fingers and toes begin to take shape.

You may feel better during the *second trimester* than you did at first. Your abdomen will expand as the baby continues to grow and you'll feel your baby begin to move before this trimester is over.

The *third trimester* can be emotionally and physically challenging as the baby is getting bigger and it is putting pressure on your organs. Signs of third trimester may include swollen ankles, backache and mounting anxiety. Your baby will likely open her or his eyes and this rapid growth may lead to more obvious fetal movements.

The *American College of Obstetricians and Gynecologists* recommends the following pregnancy terms:

Early term: between 37 weeks and 38 weeks

Full term: between 39 weeks and 40 weeks

Late term: between 41 weeks and 41 weeks

The condition before completion of 37 weeks are considered as *"Pre-term"* and events after 42 weeks are called *"Post-term"*.

During pregnancy, the health of your baby is top priority.

2) Prenatal Care

This is the medical care that is recommended for women before and during pregnancy for ensuring the good health of baby and mother. Aim of prenatal care is to diagnose potential threats early so that they can be prevented if possible. It is normally carried out by recommending an adequate diet plan, supplements intake and soft exercises etc. to make women healthy and fit.

3) Pregnancy Complications

If you are suffering from any chronic condition such as epilepsy, depression or diabetes then it could affect your pregnancy. You may require close monitoring and specific treatment plans to prevent pregnancy problems. Pregnancy complications vary as each pregnancy is different. Some are more common than others and may include: morning sickness, hyperemesis gravidarum, Indigestion, constipation, breathing difficulties, itching, piles (haemorrhoids), vaginal discharge, varicose veins, backache, pelvic ligament pain, tingling and numbness, symphysis pubis pain, and leg cramps.

Some other serious *Pregnancy complications* include:

a) Low birth weight

This is caused by poor nutrition or can be an effect of an STD, or no prenatal care. Babies who are born pre-maturely may risk blindness, respiratory infections, cerebral palsy, learning disabilities and heart infections.

b) Ectopic Pregnancy

This can be caused by an infection such as pelvic inflammatory disease. Women with reproductive disorders such as endometriosis are also at risk. It is also called "Tubal pregnancy" as egg is fertilized in the tube, outside the uterus because of a narrowing of fallopian tube. Ectopic pregnancy can cause dizziness, severe pelvic pain, heavy bleeding and even death. Methotrexate or Emergency surgery is used for the treatment.

c) Pre-term Labor

It happens when mother's body tries to deliver the baby before 37 weeks. It occurs when contractions are stronger, longer and closer. Bed rest and medications are advised to help the pregnancy go full-term in serious cases.

d) Gestational Diabetes

It develops when the mother's body is not making insulin in sufficient amounts. It usually develops in the second trimester and cannot be treated by pills only. Treatment is carried out through insulin and diet.

e) Molar Pregnancy

This is an abnormality of the placenta and happens when the egg and sperm join together at fertilization. This is a rare abnormality.

f) Rh Negative Disease

Rh factor is determined by the protein that surrounds red blood cells. A woman is considered Rh negative if the protein is absent. If the Rh negative mother conceives an Rh positive baby then she starts to produce antibodies against the Rh positive baby. Rho GAM is the medicine given at about 28 weeks and again at birth to avoid these antibodies if the baby is Rh positive.

g) Gestational hypertension

This is a condition of high blood pressure (systolic blood pressure $\geq$140 mmHg and/or diastolic blood pressure $\geq$90 mmHg) during pregnancy.

h) Chronic hypertensio

B.P over 140/90 before pregnancy, in early pregnancy (before 20 weeks) or after pregnancy.

i) Gestational Hypertension

High B.P that develops after 20 weeks in pregnancy and goes away after delivery.

j) Preeclampsia

Both Gestational and Chronic hypertension may lead to this serious condition after 20 weeks of pregnancy. *Symptoms* are protein in urine and high blood pressure.

Hypertension can prevent the placenta from getting sufficient blood that might result in less oxygen & food getting to the baby and ultimately resulting in low birth weight.

k) Miscarriage or Spontaneous abortion (SAB)

This is the term used when pregnancy ends on its own within 20 weeks of gestation. Most miscarriages happen during the first 13 weeks of gestation. The cause of a miscarriage may be different but during the first trimester the most common reason is chromosomal abnormality. Other reasons of miscarriage are infections, maternal health problems, hormonal problems, maternal age, maternal trauma, improper implantation of egg into uterine lining or unhealthy lifestyle. There are so many other possible complications during pregnancy, but all are not discussed here as it will divert us from the main topic of discussion.

l) Child birth

Child birth is the process in which the infant is born. Immediately after birth, both baby and the mother are hormonally connected i.e. the mother through the release of oxytocin that is also released during breast-feeding. Skin-to-skin contact after birth is also very beneficial to reduce baby's cries and to improve mother-baby interaction.

m) Post-natal Period

This begins immediately after the birth of the baby and it is extended to 6 weeks. In this period, the mother starts to return back to pre-pregnancy conditions including hormonal changes and change in uterus size.

n) Effects of Pregnancy on Woman with Diabetes

Below are the effects that can occur during pregnancy if a woman is diabetic:

-Delayed gastric emptying and reflux esophagitis in later pregnancy and changes in eating patterns.

-Need of close blood glucose level monitoring.

-Increased Insulin dose causing decreased Insulin sensitivity by approx. 50%.

-Risk of retinopathy.

-Risk of hypoglycemia.

-Risk of decline in renal function in pregnant woman with nephropathy.

-Decreased renal threshold to glucose, predisposing to UTIs.

o) Effects of Maternal Diabetes on Pregnancy
Below are the effects of Diabetes Mellitus that need to be addressed during pregnancy:

-Preconception counseling

-Increased risk of miscarriage

-Increased congenital malformations

-Regular monitoring and ultrasound

-Risk of preeclampsia

-Early delivery and caesarean section ratio

-Increased prenatal mortality

-Macrosomia with difficult delivery

NOTE: All these points will be discussed in further detail in this book in coming chapters under different headings.

4) Additional Concerns in Pregnancy Complicated by Gestational Diabetes Mellitus

Nausea and vomiting are the two most common complications in pregnancy, usually known as *Morning sickness.* Morning sickness is a natural but poorly understood discomfort that occurs usually in the early stages of pregnancy, around the 4th to 6th week of pregnancy. The cause of Morning sickness is not known exactly but an elevated level of the Human Chorionic Gonadotropin (HCG) hormone in the first trimester could be the reason. Other possible causes are increased levels of estrogen or decreased levels of progesterone.

Morning sickness is not harmful as women with nausea and vomiting have a decreased risk of low birth weight, spontaneous abortion, pre-term delivery, and intrauterine growth retardation. There is no specific treatment for nausea and vomiting but different steps can be taken to decrease the symptoms of nausea and vomiting.

Recommendations to alleviate the symptoms:

Small amounts of food should be consumed every 2 to 4 hours as eating a large portion of food may increase gastric motility and triggers nausea. An empty stomach can also exaggerate the symptoms of nausea and vomiting.

Sometimes, toothpaste can also trigger nausea so it is advised not to brush immediately after eating or when you wake up. Toothpaste can be substituted with Baking soda to avoid nausea.

Small snacks should be eaten before bedtime to maintain blood glycemic levels throughout the night. An early morning snack such as bread or crackers can help in maintaining blood glucose levels and to prevent nausea too.

As a general rule, liquids should be consumed between meals or 30 to 45 min after meals. Caffeinated beverages should be avoided as they increase gastric secretions and carbonated water & sugar free carbonated beverages are recommended.

Fried and greasy foods increase the gastric acidity so they must be avoided. Foods with less fat and easily digested carbohydrates are better to consume.

Cooking odors can exaggerate nausea so this should be avoided. Ginger is effective in the treatment of nausea so it can be used in food or tea, for example.

In women with GDM, nausea and vomiting can affect blood glucose levels. So, in addition to the above recommendations, these women should consume a small amount of food to avoid a drop in blood glycemic levels. Check urine ketones daily as long as the symptoms of morning sickness persist.

a) Hyperemesis Gravidarum (HG)
It is the most serious form of nausea and vomiting and is associated with ketosis, dehydration, electrolyte imbalance, and weight loss. Symptoms of HG can affect the health of pregnant mother (jaundice and coma) and the fetus (low birth weight, preterm delivery, and intrauterine growth retardation). The exact cause of HG is unknown but it is assumed that it could be due to phosphate deficiency, hyperthyroidism, thiamin deficiency, and psychological factors.

b) Management of HG
Management mainly focuses on the ways to reverse nutrition depletion and minimize nausea and vomiting. Course of treatment involves one or more of the following:

a) Traditional method: In this method, the woman is admitted to hospital and Sodium Chloride is given intravenously to treat dehydration. Solids are introduced in the diet slowly when the patient is able to tolerate the solid foods.

b) Enteral nutrition: This is used as an alternative to traditional methods when they fail. Enteral feeding is done when women are hydrated with balanced electrolyte levels.

c) Medications: The use of anti-emetics is very controversial in treating HG as some anti-emetics are taken off from the market due to their teratogenicity (e.g. Thalidomide). Medications used for treatment of HG include metoclopramide, phenothiazine, pyridoxine, chlorpromazine, prochlorperazine, meclizine, dimenhydrinate, and diphenhydramine, as they don't have any teratogenic effects.

d) Parenteral nutrition: This is used only the serious situation where inability to tolerate enteral food threatens the health of the fetus. Parenteral nutrition meets the nutrient requirements of both mother and fetus and it reverses the effects of weight loss. Each patient should be individually analyzed to determine the need of parenteral nutrition.

Chapter 3: Symptoms, Causes & Risk Factors of Gestational Diabetes

1) Causes of Gestational Diabetes

Gestational diabetes is high blood sugar (glucose) level & occurs in approximately 4% of all pregnancies.

Almost all women experience some degree of impaired glucose intolerance due to hormonal changes that occur during pregnancy. Usually the blood sugar is higher than normal, but not high enough to have diabetes. During the latter part of pregnancy (most probably; the 3rd trimester), the hormonal changes place pregnant women at risk of developing gestational diabetes.

The increased levels of certain placental hormones help shift nutrients from the mother to the developing fetus. Other placental hormones work by resisting the actions of insulin, and thus prevent the mother from developing low blood sugar.

Over the course of the pregnancy, the excess of these hormones leads to a higher blood sugar level due to progressive impaired glucose intolerance. To bring the blood sugar levels back to normal, the body makes more insulin.

To overcome the effect of pregnancy hormones on blood glucose/sugar levels, the mother's pancreas is able to produce about three times more insulin than the normal amount. If the pancreas fails to produce enough insulin, the blood sugar levels will rise, resulting in gestational diabetes.

Pregnancy is mainly characterized by insulin resistance and hyper insulinemia. Therefore, it may predispose some women to developing diabetes due to insulin resistance; this resistance takes its origin from the following;

-Placental secretion of diabetogenic hormones (growth hormone, corticotropin releasing hormone, placental lactogen, & S progesterone)

-Increased deposition of maternal adipose

-Decreased exercise

-Increased calorie intake

Along with these, a few other endocrine and metabolic changes ascertain the continuous, adequate supply of fuel and nutrients to the fetus.

GDM commonly occurs in women with pancreatic dysfunction. Thus there is an inadequate amount of insulin that is required during pregnancy to overcome the insulin resistance created by changes in diabetogenic hormones.

2) Warning signs of gestational diabetes

There may be mild or even no symptoms at all. Whatever the case is; symptoms are not life threatening to the pregnant woman. Also, the blood glucose level usually gets back to normal after delivery.

The signs and symptoms indicating GD may include:

-Blurred vision
-Weakness
-Frequent infections (in bladder, vagina or skin)
-dehydration

-Increased/frequent urination
-Nausea/vomiting
-Weight loss inspite of increase in appetite
-Sugar in urine

As there is an increased state of insulin resistance during pregnancy, which contributes to the diagnosis of gestational diabetes, it may also predispose a woman to developping stress/depression.

Hyperglycemia, a problem that occurs with gestational diabetes, has been found to have a direct relation with depression. Lower insulin sensitivity is observed in stressed patients, and insulin resistance may improve with depression therapy.

A pregnant woman may end up with high amniotic fluid levels in the presence of uncontrolled GD. Polyhydramnios is the condition diagnosed in about 10% of pregnant diabetics, most probably in their third trimester. It is a serious concern because when this extra amniotic fluid breaks, it produces a greater risk of an umbilical cord prolapse (when the cord falls through the cervical opening) or a placental abruption, both requiring an immediate c-section.

3) Risk Factors for Gestational Diabetes

Pregnant women who fulfill any one of the aforementioned criteria appear to be at an increased risk of developing gestational diabetes; however, the risk increases in the presence of multiple risk factors:

-A **positive family history** of diabetes (especially in first degree relatives)

-Body weight - Too much weight gain in early-mid pregnancy has been associated with either having one abnormal value on a 3hr GTT performed in the late 2nd trimester or GD.

-Women who weigh $\geq$110 percent of ideal body weight or have BMI >30 kg/m^2 prior to pregnancy

-Significant weight gain in early adulthood

-Weight gain between pregnancies

-Excessive gestational weight gain

-Age >25yrs

-Previous delivery of a baby >9 pounds/4kg

-Personal history of glucose intolerance

-Member of an **ethnic group** with a higher rate of type 2 diabetes (e.g., Hispanic-American, African-American, Native American, South or East Asian, Pacific Islander).

-History of giving birth to malformed infants or sudden perinatal loss

-Maternal birth-weight >9lbs/4kg or <6lbs/2.7kg

-PCO - Polycystic ovary syndrome

-Currently on glucocorticoids

-Essential hypertension or pregnancy-related hypertension

-Metabolic syndrome

4) Chances recurrence of gestational diabetes in second pregnancy

A personal history of a metabolic disorder in a previous pregnancy potentially increases the chance for a woman to have GD for the second time (either in second or third pregnancy).

A few suggested steps may be helpful in this regard to help you to prevent it and keep the risks low. Eating healthy foods, following a routine with plenty of physical activity (regular exercise), and gradual weight loss (if a woman is overweight) are some common ways that can help reduce the risk.

According to research, the chance of recurrence of GDM in the second pregnancy or for the second time is about 40-50%, which is obviously high.

If a woman who had GD during her first pregnancy is trying to conceive again, it is advised to consult a doctor first to completely understand the necessary steps needed to be taken and also to understand lifestyle changes to be adopted to the reduce risk of getting GD for the second time.

5) Is GD preventable?

A few measures may be taken to successfully reduce the risk of developing gestational diabetes. Various weight loss and exercise programs of brisk walking, stairs climbing and a few other vigorous activities before/early in pregnancy may actively reduce the risk of developing gestational diabetes in overweight women.

6) Weight loss

The benefit of weight loss can be elaborated by considering the following examples:

-In a population-based cohort study, obese women who lost at least 10lbs between pregnancies decreased the risk of GDM compared to women who had a weight loss of <10lbs.

-In a comparative study of two groups of women; comparing one who delivered before, with the other group who delivered after bariatric surgery, the incidence of GDM was found to be considerably lower in those who delivered before.

7) Exercise

As it is effective to reduce the risk of type 2 diabetes in non-pregnant individuals, likewise regular exercise lowers the risk of developing gestational diabetes.

-The worth of physical activity was further illustrated by a meta-analysis that included 7 pre-pregnancy and 5 early pregnancy studies. Women with regular/higher pre-pregnancy physical activity had approximately one half the risk of developing GDM. Physical activity in early pregnancy was also found to be protective.

-On the contrary, a meta-analysis of 3 randomized trials (n = 826 women) found no significant effect in the reduction of risks of GDM compared with routine care by setting off an exercise program during pregnancy. However, this analysis was dominated by a large trial of 702 healthy women with normal weight who underwent a 12-week exercise program beginning in 18-22 weeks of gestation, which may have accounted for the lack of desired benefit. Moreover, a randomized trial published after the meta-analysis also failed to show a reduction in GDM in women who underwent an exercise program during the 2nd trimester.

Few studies performed on the role of dietary factors in the development of GDM diabetes didn't get success to prove reduction in the risk. However, a healthy diet is helpful in weight loss.

A pilot study reported that the dietary supplement *myo*-inositol, when administered during pregnancy, reduced the risk of developing GD in a high risk population. In this open label trial, 220 non-obese gravidas at risk of gestational diabetes due to positive family history of diabetes were randomly assigned to receive *myo*-inositol (2 g twice daily) plus folic acid (400 mcg twice daily) or folic acid alone from the end of the first trimester until the date of delivery. Gestational diabetes (by IADPSG/ADAcriteria) developed in 6% of *myo*-inositol treated subjects VS 15% of control subjects. Fetal macrosomia was also reduced (0 versus 7%) & average birth weight was 162g lower in the treated group. Though promising, further studies need to be performed to establish the safety and efficacy of this intervention in the general pregnant population.

Chapter 4: How To Get Diagnosed

1) Gestational Diabetes Screening: Benefits & Harms

The process of screening is helpful to identify whether a pregnant woman has diabetes. This decreases the rate of a disease, particularly macrosomia, shoulder dystocia and preeclampsia in both mother and fetus.

Whether it is screening or a diagnostic test, both involve drinking glucose-containing drinks and/or blood glucose measurement. Although none of these tests are associated with serious, harmful maternal or fetal effects, not all women can tolerate such hyperosmolar drinks.

After diagnosis of gestational diabetes, the next step is management, which involves:

-Changes in dietary habits

-An increased frequency of prenatal visits

-Monitoring of blood glucose levels

-Insulin therapy

-Additional monitoring of mother and fetus

2) Screening versus Diagnostic Testing

Screening identifies the individuals who do not exhibit symptoms of diabetes, but who have a high probability of having or developing a specific disease. It is usually performed as a two-step process.

-Step one identifies individuals at increased risk for the disease

-Step two is diagnostic testing, which is definitive but more complicated or expensive than the screening test. Therefore, it can be limited to individuals at high risk. Alternatively, a diagnostic test can be administered to all individuals, which is a one-step process.

3) Approaches to screening

a) Two step approach

It is recommended by ACOG and is the most widely used approach for identifying pregnant women with diabetes in the United States. It consists of a screening glucose challenge test, followed by a three hour oral GTT in patients screened as positive.

b) One step approach

It is a simplified diagnostic test proposed by the IADPSG and approved by the ADA. The test is performed by a 75 gram, two hour oral GTT and requires only a single, elevated value for diagnosis. The ADA supports one-step diagnostic testing for gestational diabetes in all pregnant women (without pre-existing diabetes).

4) Who qualifies for screening?

According to the recommendations of the IADPSG, organizations from around the world are now concentrating on their criteria for screening and diagnosis of gestational diabetes.

In the United States, 90% of pregnant women have at least one risk factor for glucose impairment during pregnancy. Therefore, universal screening appears to be the most practical approach.

ACOG recommends worldwide screening for gestational diabetes. Furthermore, the publication of second randomized trial demonstrated the benefits of diagnosis and treatment of mild gestational diabetes. The USPSTF proposed in a 2013 draft statement, *"Screening for gestational diabetes mellitus (GDM) in asymptomatic pregnant women after 24 weeks of gestation is mandatory."*

5) When to screen

The screening is usually performed at 24-28 weeks of pregnancy. However, depending on a few factors (such as obesity, personal history of GDM or family history of DM and glycosuria) it may be performed as early as in the first prenatal visit, which is consistent with the IADPSG's new recommendations for diagnosis of GDM. Women with a history of GDM have a 33-50% risk of recurrence, including unrecognized inter-gestational type-II diabetes.

6) How to screen

There is no universal standard for screening and diagnosis of GDM. In the United States, the current practice is a two-step approach.

a) Two step approach

This approach begins with a challenge test (also known as one-hour GTT) for screening, where an oral loading dose of 50 gram glucose is administered. The oral glucose is given regardless of the time elapsed since the last meal. The plasma glucose is measured one hour later; a value ≥130 mg/dL is used as the threshold (because of improved sensitivity). Screening and diagnostic tests that measure glucose concentration should be performed on venous plasma using a precise enzymatic method.

For instance, in a systematic review of cohort studies of screening tests for GDM by the USPSTF;

At the 130 mg/dL (7.2 mmol/L) threshold

The sensitivity was 88-99% and Specificity 66-77% (when validated against Carpenter/Coustan and National Diabetes Data Group [NDDG] criteria for diagnosis of gestational diabetes).

At the 140 mg/dL (7.8 mmol/L) threshold

-Sensitivity was lower (70-88%), but

-Specificity was higher (69-89%) (When validated against a variety of criteria: Carpenter/Coustan, ADA, NDDG, World Health Organization [WHO], Canadian Diabetes Association [CDA]).

The oral GTT performed better than FST at a threshold of 85 mg/dL (4.7mmol/L) for identifying women who were ultimately diagnosed with GDM.

No threshold for glycated hemoglobin (A1C) had both good sensitivity and specificity as a screening test for GDM.

A1C thresholds in three studies were;

- 5.0%, sensitivity 92%, specificity 28%

- 5.3%, sensitivity 12%, specificity 97%

- 5.5% sensitivity 86%, specificity 61%, respectively

Whereas, one other used A1C 7.5% - sensitivity 82% and specificity 21%.

Based on similar findings, ACOG has stated that the oral GTT should be used for screening by using either a 140 mg/dL (7.8 mmol/L) or 130 mg/dL (7.2 mmol/L) threshold. Women with an elevated value are then given a 100 gram three-hour oral GTT for a confirmed diagnosis.

b) One step approach

The IADPSG felt that the decision of initial screening for diabetes at the first prenatal visit should be based upon the history of abnormal glucose metabolism in the population and also on the local circumstances. For universal testing, it was suggested to obtain A1C. However, this approach is not validated by data from randomized trials yet.

It is certified by the ADA but not by ACOG. As per IADPSG estimate, 18% of all pregnant women will be diagnosed with GDM. ACOG orated that the one step approach would increase health care costs.

As discussed earlier, diagnosis of evident diabetes is made in women who meet any of the following criteria at their first prenatal visit:

*Fasting plasma glucose ≥126 mg/dL [7.0 mmol/L], or

*A1C ≥6.5%, or

*Random plasma glucose ≥200 mg/dL [11.1 mmol/] that is subsequently confirmed by elevated fasting plasma glucose or A1C

According to the recommendations of ADA, a diagnosis of GDM at the initial prenatal visit can be made if the fasting plasma glucose is ≥92 mg/dL [5.1mmol/L]. In men and non-pregnant women, an A1C value ≥6.5% (≥48 mmol/mol) is one of the tests that may be used to diagnose diabetes.

If the evident or gestational diabetes has not been diagnosed with initial testing at the first prenatal visit, a 75 gram two hour oral GTT should be administered at 24 to 28 weeks of gestation to all patients.

7) Glucose Tolerance Test

The oral GTT is less accurate, but is still a practical means of diagnosing GDM. The GTT has poor reproducibility, which is evident from a study that performed two oral GTTs 1-2 weeks apart in 64 pregnant women whose 50 gram glucose challenge was greater than 135 mg/dL found that only 50/64 (78%) had reproducible test results. Nevertheless, it is a practical means of diagnosing gestational diabetes.

The GTT may be omitted in women with a markedly elevated random glucose concentration (>200 mg/dL [11.1mmol/L]) to avoid the extreme hyperglycemia in such glucose intolerant women.

a) 100 gram three-hour oral glucose tolerance test

It is generally used during pregnancy in the United States and is currently recommended by ACOG; two elevated glucose values are needed for a positive test. Carbohydrate loading for three days has been recommended before this test, provided the patient is not on a low carbohydrate diet.

b) 75 gram two-hour oral glucose tolerance test

Being more convenient, highly sensitive for identifying the pregnancy at risk and better tolerated, this is recommended by the IADPSG and ADA. Only one elevated glucose value is required and the cut-offs are somewhat lower.

This conclusion is further supported by results from the Hyperglycemia and Adverse Pregnancy Outcome (HAPO) study of more than 23,000 pregnancies evaluated with a 75 gram two hour oral GTT. The investigators found a continuum of increasing risk of adverse outcomes (including macrosomia, cesarean delivery, neonatal hypoglycemia, and preeclampsia).

The IADPSG defined thresholds for the 75 gram two hour oral GTT based on outcome data reported in the HAPO study. These thresholds represent the glucose values at which the odds of infant birth weight, cord C-peptide (proxy for fetal insulin level), and percent body fat >90 percentile were 1.75 times the estimated odds of these outcomes at mean glucose levels, based on fully adjusted logistic regression models.

8) Patients unable to tolerate Oral Hyperosmolar Glucose

a) Test alternatives to the GCT and GTT

The highly concentrated hyperosmolar glucose solution can cause gastric irritation, delayed emptying and gastrointestinal osmotic imbalance, leading to nausea and also vomiting in a small percentage of women. Better tolerated alternatives (candy, a predefined meal, or commercial soft drink solution) to the oral screening and GTT have been proposed, but appear to be less sensitive and need to be validated in large studies, as none of these are certified by either ADA or ACOG.

b) Serial glucose monitoring

For women at a high risk of GDM but intolerant to oral glucose loading dose; periodic random fasting and two-hour postprandial blood glucose testing is a good monitoring option. Women having dumping syndrome after a roux-en-Y gastric bypass procedure are unlikely to tolerate a hyperosmolar glucose solution, here also the serial glucose monitoring is useful.

c) Fasting plasma glucose

In a systematic review of cohort studies of screening tests for GDM performed for the USPSTF, in women who didn't have GDM, a fasting plasma glucose level less than 85 mg/dL (4.7 mmol/L) performed well for identifying diabetes at 24 weeks of gestation. However, the performance of a value above 85 mg/dL (4.7mmol/L) performed a bit lower compared to the oral glucose challenge test for identifying women with GDM.

d) Intravenous GTT

This is alternative for patients who are intolerant to an oral glucose load, although it is neither a standard approach nor widely used. One author (DC) has found it to be useful in patients who cannot tolerate oral glucose for testing. In this test, plasma glucose is measured at 10 and 60 minutes, and then test dose of 25gm glucose is rapidly infused intravenously. The value obtained at 10-min plasma glucose level is divided by the 60-minute glucose value to have a quotient (Q), which describes the rate of loss of glucose from the circulation. Healthy individuals will clear glucose more rapidly compared to diabetics. A table can be used to convert the Q to a K value, which represents the slope of the glucose loss curve. The lower limit of normal (mean $-$ 2 standard deviations) K values were found to be 1.37 in the first trimester, 1.18 in the second trimester, and 1.13 in the third trimester.

e) A1C

A large overlapping in the distribution of A1C values between women with normal, borderline abnormal and mildly abnormal blood glucose levels is observed. Therefore, it not a suitable choice to detect **slightly** impaired glucose tolerance. An A1C $\geq$6.5% is suggestive of type-II diabetes, and is also one of the criteria for diagnosis of overt diabetes in pregnancy proposed by the IADPSG and certified by the ADA. The data are accruing that during pregnancy, when A1C levels are a bit lower than in the non-pregnant state (in most laboratories this level is approx. 5.3%), they may identify those women at risk of delivering a large gestational age infant. However, an A1C below this level is insufficient to provide evidence against the diagnosis of diabetes and therefore cannot substitute oral GTT. In men and non-pregnant women, an A1C value of $\geq$6.5% ($\geq$48mmol/mol) is one of the tests generally used to diagnose diabetes.

Chapter 5: Pregnancy Management in GD

GDM, if undetected or not managed effectively, can cause complications. These complications associated with Gestational Diabetes can affect both the mother and the fetus.

The baby of a woman diagnosed with GDM may be at increased risk of:

-Premature birth

-Trauma during the birth

-Neonatal hypoglycemia, which may cause poor feeding, cyanosed skin and tetchiness

-High birth weight

-Early (preterm) birth and respiratory distress syndrome

-Jaundice

-Development of Type 2 diabetes or obesity later in life

-Untreated GDM can even result in a perinatal death

GDM may also increase the mother's risk of:

-Placental abruption that may cause vaginal bleeding and/or constant abdominal pain

-Induction of labour

-High blood pressure, preeclampsia and eclampsia

-Future diabetes

1) Pregnancy management in GD

The obstetrical challenges encountered while caring for a pregnant woman with GDM includes extensive knowledge of:

–   The related maternal and fetal risks

–   Antepartum maternal and fetal monitoring

–   Monitoring fetal growth and well-being via obstetrical ultrasound

–   Intelligent decisions about timing & route of delivery

–   Intrapartum obstetric & glycemic management

–   postpartum assessment.

The following content will address the issues related to obstetric management of women screened at 24-28 weeks of gestation and diagnosed with GDM.

2) Focus of Prenatal Care

In prenatal care of women with GDM, along with the routine pregnancy issues, identification and management of conditions specific to glucose impairment are focused on. Maintaining a good glycemic control is the key intervention to reduce the rate and/or severity of these conditions.

There is an increased risk of giving birth to an infant with congenital malformations or overt vasculopathy (any disease of blood vessels) in women with pre-GDM. However, it is not observed in women with GDM.

The conditions that are more common in GDM include:

3) Macrosomia

It has been consistently demonstrated in randomized trials that maternal hyperglycemia significantly increases a woman's chances of having a large fetus for gestational age (LGA) in addition to excessive maternal weight gain (>40lbs or 18 kg), which increases the risk up to two-folds. Macrosomia potentially increases the risk of operative delivery (cesarean or instrumental vaginal) and adverse neonatal outcomes (such as shoulder dystocia, fracture of clavicle and brachial plexus injury during delivery). The disproportion in the ratio of the size of the shoulder or abdomen-to-head in infants of diabetic mothers also appears to increase the risk.

a) Preeclampsia

Compared to women without GDM, the risk of preeclampsia is higher in women with GDM. This is probably due to insulin resistance. The probability is supported by the findings of several studies, which showed a significant association between mid-trimester insulin resistance and the development of preeclampsia even in the absence of GDM.

b) Hydramnios

This is an excessive accumulation of amniotic fluid, more common in women with GDM. However, it is not proven to produce a significant increase in perinatal morbidity or mortality.

c) Stillbirth

Due to poor glycemic control, the fetus of a woman with GDM appears to be at a comparatively higher risk of intrauterine demise.

d) Neonatal morbidity

There is an increased risk of metabolic disorder in the neonates of pregnancies complicated by GDM. The disorder may be either:

-Hypoglycemia

-Hyperbilirubinemia

-Hypocalcemia

-Erythremia

-Respiratory distress syndrome

e) Gestational diabetes affects on baby

The risks associated with GDM extend beyond the pregnancy and neonatal period, where GDM may affect the offspring's risk of:

-Becoming obese

-Developing glucose intolerance

-Metabolic syndrome

GDM is also an indication of the development of maternal type-2 diabetes and diabetes-associated vascular disease later on.

f) Keep up a healthy pregnancy weight

Generally, a woman should gain about 2-4lbs during the first three months of gestation and 1lb a week during the rest of pregnancy and 1 ½ pounds per week for a twin pregnancy.

In an observational study on patterns of weight gain in pregnant women with/without GDM, women with GDM gained comparatively less weight than non-diabetic women where women gained weight at a constant rate. Weight gain was influenced by BMI and country of birth.

Ideal weight gain merely depends on the pre-pregnancy weight of the woman. One should consult her doctor about his/her views on how much weight a woman should ideally gain during her entire pregnancy.

4) Pregnancy Management Guidelines

a) How good does the glucose control have to be?

Glycemic control is the keystone of management of gestational diabetes. Avoiding maternal hyperglycemia during labor reduces the risk of fetal acidosis and neonatal hypoglycemia. The risk of adverse neonatal metabolic disorder outcome is directly related to maternal hyperglycemia.

b) Antenatal fetal testing

The literature that supports antenatal fetal testing in pregnancies complicated by GDM consists primarily of observational series. Rare to no fetal losses at all were reported among a group of pregnancies followed by various testing regimens. However, there are no randomized trials that evaluate obstetrical management of women with GDM specifically, and also the findings from the small number of cohort and case-control studies are uncertain.

The practice of fetal testing is based on the severity of GDM.

The presence of other risk factors contributing to adverse pregnancy outcome, such as advanced maternal age, past history of stillbirth and the presence of co-morbid diseases like chronic hypertension must also be considered.

c) Schedule to follow

It is natural to start testing in the 3rd trimester. The frequency of the actual tests utilized varies from institution to institution and practice settings.

Generally, the specialists recommend similar management to maintain euglycemia for both women requiring insulin or an oral anti-hyper glycemic agent and women with pre-gestational diabetes or other conditions that place the pregnancy at an increased risk of adverse outcome. Such women normally undergo antenatal testing twice weekly, starting from 32 weeks of gestation. The women, who are euglycemic with nutritional therapy alone and have no other pregnancy complications, do not appear to be at increased risk of stillbirth; therefore, the ante partum fetal surveillance with non-stress testing or biophysical profile scoring is not required.

d) Assessment of fetal growth

It may be useful to identify:

-Cases where induction of labor is beneficial before the fetus grows too large

-Cases where scheduled cesarean delivery may be beneficial if fetal size exceeds some threshold

-Women with poor glycemic control

However, with regret, there is no such method of fetal growth assessment that performs well. All currently available methods are neither sensitive nor specific, especially for identifying the large size in gestational age fetuses.

The sonographical findings of a review of pregnant women with diabetes treated with insulin revealed that the estimated fetal weight had to be ≥4800 grams for there to be at least a 50% chance that the infant's birth weight would be ≥4500 grams. Studies in non-diabetic pregnancies reported similar results. Investigators have tried to find a more sensitive modality to estimate fetal weight, but there is little evidence that these experimental modalities can improve on existing two-dimensional ultrasound technology.

Considering these limitations, a wide practice spectrum has evolved. This spectrum ranges from an ultrasound at 36 weeks of gestation (for assessment of potential for macrosomia) to frequent ultrasounds (to monitor fetal growth) at 28, 32 and 36 weeks of gestation.

Any false positive finding may lead to iatrogenic (induced inadvertently by a physician or surgeon or by medical treatment or diagnostic procedures) complications, therefore, fetal growth is not monitored sonographically in euglycemic women with A1 GDM (medical nutritional therapy alone). For instance, one study reported an increase in cesarean delivery among women who had an ultrasound examination in the 3rd trimester, even after controlling birth weight.

e) Timing of delivery
Will I carry the baby to full term or deliver early?

A key issue in the management of women with GDM is to decide whether to induce labor, and if so, when?

The potential benefits of induction are:

-Avoidance of late stillbirth

-Avoidance of delivery-related complications of continued fetal growth (such as shoulder dystocia or cesarean delivery).

The potential disadvantages include:

-The risks of induction. If the induction caesarian delivery fails, tachysystole iatrogenic prematurity may occur.

The optimal timing of delivery in GDM has not been evaluated in well-designed trials. Therefore, due to inadequate data, an evidence-based recommendation cannot be made.

The only randomized trial in diabetic pregnancies included 200 women with uncomplicated insulin-requiring diabetes and appropriately grown fetuses to evaluate delivery timing. Elective induction during the 38th week of gestation was beneficial compared to expectant management because of a lower incidence of LGA infants, fewer cases of shoulder dystocia, and also a lower rate of cesarean delivery. The expectantly managed group delivered, on average, a week later where 50% of women in due course required induction for obstetrical indications.

According to the findings of a cohort study of induction of labor in women with GDM treated with insulin; the group electively induced at 38-39 weeks of gestation had a considerably lower rate of shoulder dystocia with no increased risk of cesarean delivery.

Other evidence supporting preventive labor induction comes from a study that compared birth outcomes resulting from the active management of risk in pregnancy at term (AMOR-IPAT) to the outcomes obtained from standard management.

In the AMOR-IPAT protocol, women with GDM were induced 8 days prior to their due date. In this retrospective cohort study, the actively managed group had a higher induction rate (63 VS 25.7

%) than the standard care group, and a lower cesarean delivery rate. Findings were similar for both nulliparous and multiparous subgroups. The median gestational age at delivery for the electively induced was 38.9 weeks and 40.1 weeks for a standard care group.

In a pilot randomized trial of this concept, the AMOR-IPAT exposed group had:

-A similar cesarean delivery rate as the standard care group

-A lower rate of neonatal-ICU unit admission

-A considerably higher rate of uncomplicated vaginal birth

-Lower mean adverse outcome index score.

The median gestational age at delivery for the electively induced group was 39.1 weeks and 40.0 weeks for the standard care group.

Based on this and other relevant data, many institutions are now following a practice pattern to manage pregnancies of women who remain euglycemic with diet and exercise alone. A discussion has also begun regarding the possibility of induction of labor when the woman reaches her estimated date of delivery, 40th week of gestation, and recommending elective induction when she reaches the 41st week of gestation, which thereby reduces the risks associated with post-term pregnancy.

For women with GDM, whose glucose levels are medically managed with insulin or oral agents, it is suggested to undergo induction of labor at the 39th week of gestation. Data from a retrospective cohort study of women with GDM indicates a statistically lower infant mortality rate at 39 weeks

(8.7/10,000) than the risk of stillbirth plus infant mortality with expectant management over an additional week (15.2/10,000). Pre-term delivery is not indicated in uncomplicated pregnancies with well controlled glucose levels. If a co-morbid medical condition (e.g. hypertension) is present or there is suboptimal glycemic control, induction of labor at 38 weeks of gestation is suggested, provided the fetal lung maturity is confirmed.

f) Scheduled cesarean delivery

The decision to perform scheduled cesarean delivery in order to reduce the risk of birth trauma from shoulder dystocia is debatable. It has been estimated that in non-diabetic pregnancies with an estimated fetal weight of ≥4500 grams, 443 cesareans are required to be performed to prevent one permanent brachial plexus injury. However, whether this trade-off justifies the increased risks of cesarean delivery remains unclear.

The American College of Obstetricians and Gynecologists (ACOG) practice bulletin on macrosomia suggests that, in non-diabetic patients, an elective cesarean delivery is reasonable provided the estimated fetal weight is ≥5.0 kg. However, ACOG is less clear about what to do in a setting of macrosomia due to diabetes; stating a scheduled cesarean "may be considered" in diabetic women with an estimated fetal weight of ≥4.5 kg.

The following key issues needs to be understood by the pregnant diabetics:

(1) The difficulty in accurately predicting birth-weight by any method

(2) The risks of a cesarean delivery in the current pregnancy

(3) The risks of a prior cesarean delivery on management and outcome of future pregnancies.

If a woman with an estimated fetal weight of ≥4500 grams decides to undergo a trial of labor, the labor progress must be keenly observed and closely followed. An operative vaginal delivery may be performed provided the fetal vertex has descended normally in the 2nd stage of labor. The reason for this is the higher risk of shoulder dystocia and brachial plexus injury associated with the instrumental delivery (use of a vacuum poses a higher risk than forceps).

g) Labor and delivery

Avoidance of maternal hyperglycemia reduces the risk of fetal acidosis and neonatal hypoglycemia. The risk of adverse neonatal metabolic outcomes (hypoglycemia, hyperbilirubinemia, hypocalcemia, erythremia) related to both antepartum and intrapartum maternal hyperglycemia share a directly proportional relation with the degree of maternal hyperglycemia.

Insulin requirements generally decrease during labor, as the work of labor, particularly uterine contractions, which requires energy and oral caloric intake, is typically reduced. Women with GDM who were euglycemic without insulin or oral anti-hyperglycemic drugs rarely require insulin during labor and delivery. While women who used insulin or oral anti-hyperglycemic drugs to maintain euglycemia during pregnancy may need an insulin infusion during labor and delivery to maintain euglycemia. Blood glucose measurement is checked every 2hrs during labor in these women and an insulin infusion is begun if the value rises above 120 mg/dL (6.7 mmol/L).

Compared to hypoglycemia, mild hyperglycemia is generally less morbid and easier to treat, it is therefore better to withhold long-acting insulin in favor of using an insulin infusion, as required, on women in labor.

For women undergoing scheduled cesarean delivery, insulin or anti-hyperglycemic drugs are suspended the morning of surgery and the woman is NPO (not allowed any oral intake).

5) Postpartum Management & Follow-up

Women with GDM should be able to resume a regular diet after delivery. At this stage, the hyperglycemic effects from placental hormones dissipate rapidly and women almost immediately revert back to the pre-pregnancy glycemic control. However, since some women with GDM may have undiagnosed type 2 DM, blood glucose concentrations (fasting and random) are monitored for 24 hours after a vaginal delivery and 48 hours after a cesarean delivery. The fasting venous glucose levels below 126 mg/dL (7 mmol/L) after delivery in women with GDM can be counseled to continue to follow a healthy diet intake, regular exercise, and achieve a healthy weight to prevent future diabetes. For elevated blood glucose concentrations, the continuance of monitoring and therapy is necessary. Postpartum depression is more common among women with diabetes (pre-gestational or gestational) compared to non-diabetic women.

6) Contraception

Any type of contraception is acceptable, provided its use is not medically contraindicated. Options in breastfeeding women on anti-hyperglycemic therapy are discussed separately.

In a study of breastfeeding Hispanic women with recent GDM, the use of progestin-only pills was associated with an increased risk of developing type 2 diabetes; however, whether the same applies to non-Hispanic women remains unclear.

In another study, depo-medroxy progesterone acetate (DMPA) use was associated with an increased risk of developing diabetes that the authors attributed to use in women with increased baseline diabetes risk, weight gain during use, and use with high baseline triglycerides and/or during breast-feeding. It is unlikely that the low systemic progesterone level related to the use of a levonorgestrel-releasing intrauterine contraceptive would produce a similar effect. If a patient is apprehensive about these hormonal issues, a copper-releasing intrauterine contraceptive is an acceptable alternative.

7) Follow-up

More than 90 percent of women with GDM revert back to normal glycemic controls after delivery. However, there is a risk of recurrent GDM, and development of glucose intolerance or overt diabetes later in life. Therefore, at least 6 weeks after delivery, an oral GTT test using a 2-hour 75 gram should be performed.

Chapter 6: Medical Treatments

High-risk pregnancy is either due to a preexisting health condition or due to any condition a woman develops during pregnancy. For this reason there is a greater chance of pregnancy complications. A high risk pregnancy needs extra monitoring and perhaps added treatment to make sure that everything goes smoothly with maternal and fetal health during pregnancy.

Gestational diabetes is usually diagnosed as a result of a screening test performed during pregnancy. If the blood sugar tests reveal high levels, the patient will be asked to go in for complete check-up immediately. In addition, the concerned doctor will schedule more-frequent, regular prenatal visits to closely monitor the course of pregnancy.

An appointment can be brief but often there are a lot of things to discuss. It is therefore a good idea to prepare ahead of time. The following information will help you know what to expect from the doctor:

1) Things to do

-Beware of pre-appointment restrictions. You need to have an empty stomach (fasting state) for a blood test.

-Pen down symptoms you're experiencing and key personal information. Although GDM often doesn't cause notable symptoms, it's better to keep a record of anything atypical that you observe, including any major trauma or recent changes in lifestyle

-Enlist all medications that you are taking, including OTC (over the counter) drugs and vitamins or supplements

-Bring along a family member or friend. Usually it is difficult to fully understand the information provided during the visit. Thus, someone who goes with you may remember the things you might have missed or forget.

2) Ask your doctor

Bring with you a list of questions. Enlist the questions in a chronological order from most important to least.

For GDM, a few basic questions one should ask the doctor include:

What measures should be adopted to help control the condition?

To suggest a dietitian or a diabetes educator to help you plan meals, exercise program, and other coping strategies

What are the warning signs/symptoms that require seeking medical attention?

Ask for take-away brochures or other printed material that will assist you in maintaining a healthy routine

In addition to the pre-planned questions, you should not hesitate to ask the doctor to clarify the things you did not understand.

3) What to expect from the doctor

The doctor will also question the patient with GDM, especially if it is the first visit. Be ready to respond, so that you may free up time to focus on other important points you want to discuss in detail.

The common questions your doctor may ask include:

Any increase in thirst or excessive urination? If yes, when did the symptoms start and how frequently?

Are there any other unusual symptoms present?

Do you have any other family member (parent or sibling) diagnosed with diabetes?

Is it your first pregnancy? If not, did you have GDM during any previous pregnancy?

Did you have any other notable problems/complications in earlier pregnancies?

If you have children, how much did each of them weigh at birth?

Have you experienced a lot of weight gain/loss at any time throughout your life?

4) Things you can do meanwhile

As soon as you are diagnosed with GDM, you can take a few steps to control it with healthy choices, such as:

If the doctor advises further evaluation, make sure to visit and follow-up appointments as soon as possible

Strictly follow the doctor's advice

Eat healthily and take time to learn about gestational diabetes

5) The Treatment Strategies

The primary goal of treatment is to keep blood sugar levels within the normal range during the pregnancy, and to ensure the good health of the fetus.

Monitoring during pregnancy

The health care provider closely checks/monitors the mother and fetus throughout the pregnancy. The fetal monitoring includes checking the health and size of the fetus.

Increased prenatal visits

Women who develop GDM have more frequent prenatal visits compared to non-GDM women (e.g. 1-2 visits every week), especially if the patient is on insulin. The purpose of these visits is to monitor the health of mother and fetus. It is quite common practice to change the dose of insulin as the pregnancy progresses.

Monitoring blood sugar levels

While you're pregnant, the health care team may advise you to check and monitor your blood sugar 4-5 times per day (starting with fasting in the morning and then randomly after meals)

This makes sure that the sugar level stays within a healthy range. Initially, it may sound inconvenient or difficult, but it gets easier with practice. It is quite simple to test the blood sugar - draw a drop of blood from your finger by using a pricking needle (lancet). Place the drop of blood on a test strip that is pre-inserted into a glucometer (a device to measure and display blood sugar levels).

The associated health care team not only monitors but also manages blood sugar levels during labor and delivery. If the blood sugar level rises, there is a release of high levels of insulin from fetus, which causes hypoglycemia (low blood sugar level) in baby exactly after birth.

A follow-up blood sugar test is equally important. After having GDM, a woman is at increased risk of developing type-2 diabetes down the line; however, maintaining a healthy lifestyle (such as a healthy diet and regular physical activity) can help reduce the associated risks.

Healthy diet & regular physical activity

Eating the right kind and appropriate quantity of food is an ideal way to control blood sugar levels. It is never advised to lose weight during pregnancy (because the body is working hard enough to support the growing baby). Instead, the doctor helps to set weight gain goals, if required. Excessive weight gain is not desirable and can lead to a higher risk of complications.

A healthy diet spotlights on fruits, vegetables and whole grain foods that are nutritious, high in fiber and low in fat & calories. Highly refined carbohydrates and sweets intake should be limited. It is recommended to consult a dietitian (regd.) or a diabetes educator to create a diet plan considering:

-Current weight

-Pregnancy weight gain goal

-Blood sugar

-Physical activities

-Food preferences and budget.

Regular physical activity undoubtedly plays a vital role in every woman's wellness plan (prior to, during and also after pregnancy) It lowers blood sugar by stimulating the body to shift glucose into cells, where it is used for energy. In addition, it increases the cells' sensitivity to insulin. Furthermore, regular physical activity helps relieve some common distresses of pregnancy, including backache, swelling and cramps in muscles, constipation and sleep disorder.

As soon as the doctor advises, aim for moderate-vigorous exercise. Those who have been inactive for a while should start slowly and then build up gradually.

Medication

Where diet and exercise are insufficient to produce desirable results, one may need insulin injections to lower blood sugar levels. Between 10-20% of women with GDM need insulin to reach the desired blood sugar levels.

A few doctors prescribe an oral medication such as glyburide to control blood sugar levels. However, others feel theres needs to be more research carried out to ascertain the safety and efficacy of injectable insulin in controlling GDM.

Additional tests to see how your baby is developing:

a) Repeated Ultrasounds

Close monitoring of baby is an important part of the treatment plan. The doctor may monitor the fetal growth and development with repeated ultrasounds or other tests, if required. If a woman doesn't go into labor by her due date, the doctor may induce labor. This is because delivering after your due date can increase the maternal and fetal risk of complications.

b) Non-stress testing

Extra tests monitor the health of the baby during the last trimester of pregnancy may be needed, especially if:

-Blood sugar levels have been high

-She is using insulin

-She experiences any pregnancy-related complications (e.g., high blood pressure)

The most commonly used test is the "Non-stress test." It is a very simple and painless test, performed after 28 weeks of gestation to monitor the fetal health to show signs of distress to the fetus, if it is not getting enough oxygen for example.

To perform the non-stress test, a belt is positioned in the region of the mother's belly to measure the fetal heart rate (response to its movement). A machine (electronic fetal monitor) placed on the abdomen hears and displays fetal heartbeat. The health care provider then compares the pattern of fetal heart rate to movements. This helps to find out whether the fetus is doing well or not.

c) Breast-feeding

Breast-feeding, if it fits with your work schedule and other obligations, may help to achieve post-pregnancy weight goals and also avoid later development of type 2 diabetes.

d) Action steps

No single thing can guarantee the prevention of gestational diabetes; however, the more healthy habits one adopts before pregnancy the better. If you have ever had gestational diabetes, the following healthy choices may your reduce risk of having it for a second time in future pregnancies or the risk of developing type-2 diabetes later in life:

- Take foods that are high in fiber but with lower fat and calories (Focus more on vegetables, fruits and whole grains)

- Do your best to have a mixture and variety of food to help you achieve goals without compromising on taste/nutrition

- Keep yourself active; regular exercise before and during pregnancy helps protect against developing GDM

- Every step you take counts and increases the chances of a healthy life. Plan 30 minutes of regular, moderate activity on most days of the week. Alternatively, several shorter sessions can be equally as good and effective.

- If you are trying to get pregnant - losing excess pounds beforehand can help you to have a healthy pregnancy.

Chapter 7: Living GD-Free

Gestational diabetes mellitus (GDM) is defined as glucose intolerance first discovered during pregnancy. It predicts the risk for overt diabetes in women. The prevalence of GDM ranges from 1.1-25.5% of pregnancies in the United States, which is influenced by diagnostic criteria and population characteristics (such as ethnicity). The incidence of GDM has increased over the past few decades in parallel with the increasing rates of obesity and type-2 diabetes mellitus. GDM is treatable, and the best treatment outcomes result from careful management and also control of blood sugar levels to optimal level. The best way to control GDM is early diagnosis and initiating treatment quickly.

Treating GDM is essential even if there are mild or no symptoms at all. It greatly reduces health problems for mother and baby.

Unfortunately, the incidence of GDM is increasing. It accounts for 90% of cases of DM in pregnancy, and shares strong association with adverse pregnancy outcomes.

As discussed in previous chapters, untreated GDM may lead to various complications, such as fetal hyper insulinemia, increased weight at birth, higher rate of cesarean deliveries, shoulder dystocia and neonatal hypoglycemia. Additionally, it is also associated with concomitant preeclampsia in pregnant woman.

Given that GDM may have long-term pathological consequences for both mother and child, it is essential to diagnose it properly and manage it correctly. Treatment of GDM is aimed to maintain euglycemia and involves:

-Regular glucose monitoring

-Dietary modifications

-Physical activity

-Lifestyle changes and sometimes

-Pharmacotherapy (where Insulin therapy is the first choice of treatment)

For women receiving pharmacotherapy, scheduled monitoring of fetal well-being with antenatal tests should be followed.

Maintaining glycemic control leads to improved pregnancy outcomes, including:

- Decrease in macrosomia

- Clinical neonatal hypoglycemia

- Cesarean section rates

The Hyperglycemia and Adverse Pregnancy Outcome trial (HAPO), a large observational trial, found that a fasting glucose level of > 105 mg/dL compared to < 75 mg/dL is associated with a 5-fold increase in risk of macrosomia.

Although lower glucose levels were associated with better primary outcomes, there were no evident thresholds at which the risks actually increased.

A report commissioned by the U.S. Preventive Services Task Force in 2008 demonstrates that treatment of women with mild GDM diagnosed after 24 weeks' gestation improved both maternal and neonatal health outcomes.

Specifically, on the basis of a single study, they found a reduction in perinatal complication such as:

- Shoulder dystocia

- Bone fracture

- Nerve palsy

This study also found less depression and a trend to better quality of life three months after parturition and also reduced maternal hypertension in the treated group.

1) Health outcomes of women with GDM

This section is about the health outcomes of woman with GDM and their offspring compared to those who do not have it.

Many first-class studies have evaluated maternal and fetal outcomes among women with untreated GDM compared to those without GDM. Although the studies employed different diagnostic criteria, the findings have been consistent.

In terms of the maternal outcomes, studies revealed that a diagnosis of GDM increases the risks of:

- Cesarean delivery

- Preeclampsia

- Gestational hypertension

Whereas, in terms of fetal outcomes, methodologically strong studies revealed a continuous directly proportional relationship between increasing glucose levels and incidence of large-for-gestational age infants and also infants with macrosomia.

In addition to this, a consistently higher risk of shoulder dystocia has been found among women with a diagnosis of GDM. Shoulder dystocia may lead to rare but important outcomes (such as brachial plexus injury).

Some studies report neonatal hypoglycemia and hyperbilirubinemia among neonates born to women suffering with GDM; however, the evidence supporting these associations has not been consistent. A strong relationship between GDM and childhood obesity has been found in a few studies. The effect on longer term outcomes in the offspring, including type 2 diabetes mellitus, remains unclear.

The Hyperglycemia and Adverse Pregnancy Outcomes (HAPO) study demonstrated that the magnitudes of maternal and fetal risks increase with the severity of maternal hyperglycemia. The HAPO study evaluated glucose tolerance at 24-32 weeks during pregnancy in more than 25,000 pregnant women from 15 centers in 9 different countries, providing information on a heterogeneous, multinational, ethnically diverse group of women.

For women with less severe hyperglycemia during pregnancy, increasing maternal glucose levels were related to:

- Increased infant birth weight

- Increase in body fat and cord C-peptide

- Increased primary cesarean delivery rate

In addition, women with GDM also had increased risks of:

- Premature delivery

- Preeclampsia

- Shoulder dystocia or birth injury

- Hyperbilirubinemia

Neonatal hypoglycemia and admissions to neonatal-ICU were more common in infants born to women diagnosed with GDM.

2) Treatment modifies the health outcome of mothers with GDM

Very few but well-designed and high-quality studies have attempted to approximate the benefits of treatment of GDM compared to no treatment. The successful treatment options included:

-Self-blood glucose monitoring

-Pharmacotherapy

-Nutrition therapy

3) Maternal Outcomes

Treatment of GDM reduced the risk of hypertensive disorders of pregnancy by approximately 40%.

The risk of shoulder dystocia was reduced by approximately 60%; however, as shoulder dystocia was a rare event, the absolute risk changed from only 3.5%(untreated) to 1.5%(with treatment)

Another consistent finding among the studies was that the treatment of GDM did not increase the risk of cesarean delivery.

4) Fetal, Neonatal, and Child Outcomes

A pooled meta-analysis of 5 randomized clinical trials found a 50% reduction in macrosomia in infants born to mothers treated for GDM.

Similarly, the randomized trials demonstrated that infants of mothers treated for GDM were less likely to be large for gestational age (absolute risk reduction was 6%).

5) Risk factors connected to gestational diabetes mellitus (GDM)

The notable risk factors connected to GDM are as follows:

- Older age

- Family history and previous history of GDM

- Obesity (Overweight)

- Polycystic ovary syndrome (PCOS)

- Hypertension

6) Potential indicators which tell whether you are at high risk for GDM

According to the American Diabetes Association, a woman may be considered at a higher risk of GDM (and requires to be screened early) if she is:

-Obese (body mass index-BMI >30)

-Had GDM in a previous pregnancy

-Has sugar in her urine

-Has a strong positive family history of diabetes

Some practitioners may screen a woman early if other risk factors also exist, such as:

-Given birth to a big baby in thr past

-History of unexplained stillbirths

-History of giving birth to a baby with a birth defect

Another study published in March's 2010 issue of *"Obstetrics & Gynecology"* found a strong association between excessive weight gain during pregnancy (particularly in the 1st trimester) and the risk of GDM. Researchers found the risk highest in obese women and in black women.

The point to remember is that many women who develop GDM don't have any risk factors. Therefore, practitioners prescribe screening at 24-28th week of gestation.

A small group of women might be considered at such a lower risk that they do not even need to get tested. You may be a part of this group if you:

-Are younger than 25

-Have ideal weight (according to height and age)

-Do not belong to any racial or ethnic group with a high prevalence of diabetes

-Have a negative family history of diabetes

-Have never had hyperglycemia

-Have no history of excessively large babies or any other pregnancy complication (usually associated with GDM).

Chapter 8: How Can I Manage My GD?

One of the best ways to stay healthy with diabetes is to control the sugar/glucose level in blood. Although, controlling diabetes can be hard at times, but keeping the blood sugar levels as close to normal as possible will surely help prevent the associated problems and further complications.

It's never too late to get the benefits of exercise, as it simply makes the person feel good. Increased physical activity during pregnancy lowers blood glucose levels and may prevent both GDM and possibly later-onset Type-2 Diabetes. According to one latest clinical trial, a moderate physical activity program performed thrice a week during pregnancy was found to improve the levels of maternal glucose tolerance in healthy, pregnant women. Also, higher levels of physical activity before/during pregnancy significantly reduces the risk of developing GDM.

While you exercise, the body uses two different sources of fuel to produce energy; sugar and free fatty acids. The sugar/glucose comes from the blood, liver and the muscles, where it is stored in the form of glycogen. During the first 15min of exercise, a considerable amount of sugar comes from either the blood stream or the muscle glycogen to produce fuel. Later on, the fuel starts coming from the glycogen present in the liver; whereas after 30 mins of exercise, the body then begins to obtain more of energy from the free fatty acids, resulting in the depletion of sugar levels and also glycogen stores.

The replacement of these glycogen stores may take 4-6hrs and even 12-24hrs with more intense activity. This rebuilding of glycogen stores puts a person with diabetes at a higher risk of developing hypoglycemia.

1) Exercise

According to ACOG recommendations, the pregnant woman needs to perform 30 minuntes or more of moderate exercise daily. The American Diabetes Association recommends initiating/continuing a program of moderate exercise in women without medical or obstetrical contraindications.

2) Recommended forms of exercise

The most suitable exercises recommended to do during pregnancy and the postpartum period include:

-Low-impact aerobics

-Swimming

-Stationary cycling

-Brisk walking

-Swiss ball exercises

-Yoga

-Light weights

-Resistant band exercises

Each exercise session should start with a 5-10 min warm-up period involving flexibility exercises (stretching) to reduce the risk of musculoskeletal injury during the workout, followed by a calm down period at the end of the exercise. In inactive women who decide to exercise during pregnancy, ACOG recommends that exercise heart rates should be ≤ 140bpm.

Exercise increases the insulin sensitivity of muscle glucose transportation and also enhances insulin action in extra-muscular tissues.

The 3 endocrine responses to exercise include:

a) A decline in plasma insulin level

b) An augment in sympathetic nervous activity causing changes in insulin counter-regulatory hormones

c) Hormones affecting sodium & water balance

The increased absorption of insulin during exercise leads to a potential increase in insulin levels, causing inhibition of the normal hepatic glucose production and at the same time muscle glucose uptake is also increased. The combined effect can produce hypoglycemia.

Prior to starting a regular exercise program, all diabetics are advised to undergo a medical assessment. Be educated on the benefits vs risks of exercise, and be aware of the potential effects exercise can have on glucose levels. During any physical activity, muscles consume glucose at a rate of 2-3 mg/kg of body weight/minute of exercise. An exercise program should be started when the glucose levels are adequately controlled.

Exercise regimes somewhat vary for each type of diabetes and according to the patients exercise habits before pregnancy.

a) Type 1 diabetic patients need to be monitored closely for exercise-induced hypoglycemia. If they exercised regularly before getting pregnant, they are supposed to be able to continue exercise during pregnancy.

2) Type 2 diabetic patients may start/continue exercise depending on preconception exercise habits. Inactive individuals who wish to begin exercising should do so after consulting a physician, starting with a low-intensity program. The progress in intensity/duration should be slow and as tolerated; maximally a 10% increase per week.

Patients need to be well aware of the warning signs; when to stop exercise and seek medical attention.

Follow these easy steps to get started:

3) Make a Plan

The beginners should ask the doctor which exercise is appropriate for them. Inquire if you need to adjust anti-diabetic medicine before you beat the track.

Next is to think about is which activity will you most likely stick with? For instance, a few suggestions are:

-Brisk walk; outdoors/indoors (either on a track or in a mall)
-Join a dance class
-Cycling; either outdoor or on a stationary bike
-Swimming; water aerobics
-Stretching
-Playing tennis
-Join aerobics or another fitness class
-Gardening
-Training with lighter weights or elastic bands.

4) How does it work?

During the moderate exercise (like walking) which makes the heartbeat a little faster, our muscles use more glucose/sugar in the blood stream. With the passing of time, this can lower blood sugar levels. Moreover, it makes the insulin in the body work better. These benefits stay for hours after the walk/workout.

The only thing to remember is that you don't need to exaggerate. Tough exercise can sometimes cause the body to make more stress hormones, which increases blood sugar temporarily after stopping exercise.

5) Set a Schedule

The best time to exercise may be after a meal; however, you should consult your doctor to help you decide what time of day is best specifically for you.

To stay motivated, you may ask a friend or family member to come along and join classes with you.

6) Getting Ready

Wear secure, comfortable shoes and cotton socks that don't pat. The right footwear is of prime importance to prevent blisters that could otherwise become serious infections for people with diabetes.

Test blood sugar before a walk/workout. Watch out, if it's below 100 consult your doctor.

Drink plenty of water before, during & after the workout.

Always remember to wear a diabetes ID necklace or bracelet while exercising.

7) The health benefits

Physical activity has many benefits in diabetics, as they are at greater risk of other complications in the long run, including cardiac problems, kidney diseases, and nerve or eye damage.

Exercise may help to cut down the risks of these diseases as well. Regular exercise leads to:

Controlled blood sugar levels

Lower blood pressures

Lowers bad (LDL) cholesterol

Elevates *good* (HDL) cholesterol

Improve circulation

Weight loss (if obese)

Reduced stress levels

Provides more energy

Strengthened heart, muscles & bones.

An increase in general physical activity is also helpful, such as taking the stairs instead of the escalator, get up and change the TV channels instead of using a remote control and other things you can do in daily life.

8) How much exercise I should do?

It is possible to reduce the need for diabetes medication if you stick with exercise. Ideally, it should be about 30 minutes every day. If not possible, then it can be divided into 3x10 minutes session each.

9) Intensity of the exercise

There is no need to exhaust yourself to get the benefits of exercise. It is advised to aim for moderate intensity. At first, physical activity may not feel good, particularly if you are obese, and a specialized exercise program may be required.

10) Monitoring Glucose Levels

People with diabetes need to be more careful while they exercise. It is recommended to always test blood sugar before starting to workout. The test has to be repeated again during and after exercise as well. This helps to observe the effect of physical activity on your body.

Glucose has potential for being a co-teratogen or teratogen surrogate because of the connection between A1C levels early in pregnancy and the prognostic malformation risks for the fetus.

Self-monitoring of blood glucose is essential during pregnancy, and patients with type 1 diabetes should especially monitor it closely.

Uncontrolled glycemia results in an increase of maternal-fetal transfer of glucose and amoni acids and also fetal hyper-inculimeia.

The metabolic changes can lead to difficult delivery due to the development of macrosomia, an increased rate of cesarean section, and an increase in fetal morbidity. Performing glucose tests at bedtime and in the morning can assist in diagnosing noctural hypoglycemia.

The purpose of self-monitoring is to detect glucose levels that are elevated to concentrations that may increase perinatal mortality. Blood glucose target in patients with GDM vary in the medical literature.

The 4th International Conference on GDM recommended maintaining the following capillary blood glucose values:

-Preprandial glucose <95mg/dl
-1hr postprandial glucose <140mg/dl, and
-2hr postprandial glucose <120mg/dl
The ACOG guidelines are the same except the 1hr postprandial glucose value, which is considered acceptable at either 130 or 140mg/dl. The 3hr, 100gm glucose tolerance test is used to

diagnose GDM. The diagnosis is confirmed if two or more plasma glucose levels meet/exceed following thresholds:

* Fasting glucose 95mg/dl

* 1hr glucose of 180mg/dl

* 2hr glucose of 155mg/dl or

* 3hr glucose of 140mg/dl

Postprandial glucose plays vital role in macrosomia. Simpson & Kast propose that maternal and neonatal outcomes in women with GDM are analogous to those in women without GDM when 2-hr postprandial glucose levels are maintained up to 144mg/dl.

It is very important to be familiar with safe blood sugar levels for exercise when taking insulin or any other medications to treat diabetes. Exercise is not at all recommended if the blood sugar is too low or too high.

Patients should avoid exercising when their insulin is at peak level.

The urine should be tested for ketones if the glucose level is > 250 mg/dl. In case of urine positive for ketones, exercise should be rescheduled. However, if the ketones are negative but the glucose level is >300mg/dl, cautions should be taken while exercising.

11) Hypoglycemia

Physical activity relates directly to blood glucose levels. However, if these levels drop too low, a low blood sugar reaction called hypoglycemia may occur.

Symptoms of hypoglycemia are:

- Feeling unstable
- Weakness
- Vertigo
- Irritability

12) Hyperglycemia

Exercise should be avoided if blood glucose levels are too high (hyperglycemia). A high blood sugar level causes the body to break down fat to make up for the missing insulin. This process produces ketones, which are dangerous compounds. Exercise is forbidden if someone is positive for ketones.

Most doctors recommend avoiding exercise with hyperglycemia. The volume reduction from osmotic diuresis may cause orthostatic changes, predisposing patients to injuries. Patients should, therefore, always carry some readily digestible carbohydrate rich food and inject glucagon if they experience hypoglycemia.

13) Tips

Always consult a doctor before starting any exercise program. The doctor will offer safe exercise options after complete evaluation. The complications, if present along with diabetes, may limit the exercise options available. For instance, if someone has nerve damage in their feet, the doctor may advise swimming instead of walking.

The time duration should be increased slowly and gradually. To begin with, it should be not more than 5-10 minutes at a time and work up to a total of 30 minute session.

Examine your feet after each workout and notice the sores or blisters, if any. Always wear comfy, well-fitted shoes to lessen the risk of foot problems.

Drink plenty of water to prevent dehydration.

Use a pedometer and aim for 10,000 steps per day (or determine whichever suits you best).

Generally, the target is 30 min aerobic activity at least 5 days a week. However, it may take you some time to get there if you've been sedentary for a long time. In such cases, medicine and diet are the preferred choice to get the level of blood sugar down and then start-up with short (5-10-minute) walks. These activities can be increased later.

14) Warning Signs
Warning Signs to Stop Exercise & Seek Medical Assessment

Exercise programs of moderate intensity have been shown to lower maternal glucose concentration in women with GDM. Whether exercise impacts on any neonatal complications is waiting for clinical trials.

Patients must be taught to palpate the uterus during exercise to detect contractions. The exercise has to be discontinued if contractions occur.

The physiological changes that occur during pregnancy produce a change in the point of gravity (lordosis), an increase in elastin and also edema (amassing of interstitial fluids).

These changes in the physiology increase the risk of soft tissue injuries at some stage in exercise.

Thus, you should consider these potential injuries and the exercises should be designed to prevent them as well as to strengthen other areas (including abdominal and lower back muscles).

To prevent aorto-caval compression & hypotension, exercise in the supine position should be avoided after the first trimester.

Exercise heart rates should be $\leq$140 bpm or 60-70% of Vo_{2max}

A meal should be consumed 1-3hrs before exercise because during exercise there is special carbohydrate consumption.

Ideally, insulin should be administered in the abdomen 1hr before exercise and should not be injected into the extremities.

Chapter 9: Meal Plans & Diet

Food can be divided into 3 nutrient groups:

-Carbohydrates

-Meat or meat substitutes

-Fats

Carbohydrates are found in grains, fruits, vegetables, and also low-fat milk. These are healthy foods which provide fiber, energy, vitamins and minerals. However, the carbohydrate consumption should be limited in case of gestational diabetes (GDM), because the type and amount of carbohydrates does matter. Eating too many or the wrong type of carbohydrate can potentially raise blood sugar levels.

1) The Basics of Carbohydrate counting

Counting carbohydrates in the foods we eat can really help to control the blood glucose. The reason for this is that carbohydrates raise blood glucose more compared to any other nutrient.

The balance between the amount of carbohydrate intake and insulin determines how much the blood glucose level can go up after a meal. This clearly means that we need to know what foods contain carbohydrates and how many carbohydrate servings one needs to eat to maintain optimum blood glucose level.

2) Why is carbohydrate counting vital in GDM management? Actually, carbohydrates and insulin are a balancing act. When a

person has diabetes, it is essential to pay close attention to the amount of carbohydrate intake. This is because carbohydrate is a nutrient that breaks down to sugar after being digested in the body. The human body uses carbohydrates for energy. For the utilization of this energy, insulin must be available to transport sugar/glucose into cells. In diabetics, there is impaired insulin production and/or utilization, where the sugar builds up in the blood, ultimately causing hyperglycemia if too much carbohydrate is taken at a time.

Therefore, counting the grams of carbohydrate in food is significant and helps to control diabetes further.

There are numerous ways in which women with GDM can manage their food intake to keep the blood glucose/sugar within the target range. Among these methods is carbohydrate counting.

3) Benefits of counting carbohydrates
Counting carbohydrates is a virtuous solution in GDM. This makes it easier to fit a wide variety of foods into a diet plan. Another great benefit is that it brings tighter control over glucose reading. This method is equally useful in cases where more intensive methods of adjusting insulin are used to control diabetes.

4) How to Use Carbohydrate Counting
The 1st step is to have a diet plan. Step-II involves learning carbohydrate containing food groups. For that, there are 3 main ways to learn about carbs in foods:

-Food choice list from dietitian

-Learn reading the nutrition facts label

-Purchase a food counts book

5) Measuring tools helpful in carbohydrate counting

Be accurate with the portion sizes of foods you eat. Invest in a food scale to weigh and try using cups to measure cereals or rice and even pasta and carb-containing beverages. Ideally, the amount of carbohydrates in each meal should remain consistent (except during insulin therapy). Carbohydrates are often at the center of a healthy diet for   a woman with   GDM.   These are nutrients that are very important for both mother and baby. It is wise to avoid foods that contain little nutritional value. In some women, blood glucose/sugar levels continue to be high, despite of healthy eating and regular physical activity. No matter if this happens, it is important not to cut back on carbohydrates because the fetus requires carbohydrates as its main source of energy.

6) A few things to know about carbohydrates and a healthy diet:

Some women with GDM may need to eat fewer carbohydrates than before getting pregnant to lower the total amount of carbohydrates, while, other women with GDM may need to avoid high sugar foods to keep the carbohydrate levels in line. However, inadequate consumption of carbohydrate may also cause problems. Therefore, most of the healthcare providers advise women with GDM to follow a plan of meals to ensure adequate, appropriate nutrition.

7) Develop a Meal Plan

Carbohydrates have the greatest effect on blood glucose. It is helpful to plan meals by balancing carbohydrates; this will surely help to maintain blood glucose levels within the target range. Also, track the carbohydrate grams or carbohydrate choices that you have consumed in the meal. For instance, look at the following calculations:

15 grams carbohydrate = 1 carbohydrate choice. Therefore, 30 grams carbohydrate = 2 choices, 45 grams carbohydrate = 3 choices, and so on.

The aforementioned chart can help determine carbohydrate choices wherever amounts are not in 15-gram increments.

8) Types of meal plans

The meal plan may be specific and gives a definite amount for each meal or snack, or it can be more general, with a total of daily carbohydrates. However, a slightly different version of the meal plan can also be made, where the grams of carbohydrates is represented as points. Recommendations for meal planning:

-Eat a balanced diet that includes a variety of food

-Eat a healthier diet; limit intake of sweets, fats, and salt

-Increase fiber intake

-Eat at the same time each day

-Try eating the same amount of carbohydrates regularly. A meal plan is something that gives a clear description of amounts and also the type of carbohydrate foods eaten at meal time. The meal plan helps maintain normal blood glucose levels, provides adequate nutrition to both mother and fetus, and prevents excessive weight gain as well. Blood glucose can be controlled well by making only a few changes to the food choices.

Some women will not respond to nutrition therapy alone and will require medications to control blood sugar/glucose level.

9) Essential components of a Meal Plan

-Maintain a minimum of 175gm carbohydrate (12 carbohydrate choices) per day which makes approx. 700 kcals from carbohydrates

-Utilize diet history to create a meal plan

-Smaller meals should contain 15-30gm carbohydrate and larger meals 45-60gm carbohydrate

-Split carbohydrate-containing food into smaller but frequent meals that are evenly spaced throughout the day. This enables the pancreas to secrete adequate amounts of insulin which then:

*Prevents the need for medication

*Minimizes hunger

*Decreases ketones in the urine

*Prevents heartburn and nausea

-Take a break at least two hours between meals to allow for 2hr postprandial blood glucose levels

-Do not allow more than 10-12hrs between dinner and the next morning meal

-It is good to consider including a small snack at bedtime. Doing so helps prevent ketone formation

-Use a record to track food and beverage intake

10) Pay Special Attention to the Breakfast Meal

Blood glucose levels may be elevated in the morning due to an increase in hormones that counter insulin's action and also because of the inadequate amounts of insulin to suppress the

87

liver's production of glucose during the night. Thus, the large amounts of carbohydrate foods at breakfast may increase the already elevated blood glucose level. Carbohydrate foods usually are less tolerated at breakfast when compared to any other meal. The following suggestions may be helpful in maintaining normal blood glucose levels at breakfast:

• Limit carbohydrate count to 15-30gm (1-2 carbohydrate choices)

• Avoid foods high in carbohydrate content

• Prefer protein enriched breakfast items

• Drink water instead of fruit juices

• To make sure that the plan is working well; monitor blood glucose response to unsweetened cereals and fruits

While planning a meal; aim for about 3 servings at each meal and 1 at each snack, where a single serving is approx. 15gm carbohydrates.

Chapter 10: Understanding The Role of Medication

Once GDM has been diagnosed in a woman, a decision needs to be made as to whether she should be treated and for how long. As little time is usually remaining from the time of the GDM diagnosis to the delivery of the baby, it is important to recognize that any unnecessary delay in therapy may result in irreversible adverse outcomes, which are truly undesirable.

Basically the treatment for GDM encompasses 3 different therapies:

-Dietary changes

-Exercise/Physical activity

-Pharmacotherapy

In cases where the patients are unable to achieve euglycemia with diet and exercise, pharmacotherapy with insulin is then recommended.

1) Medical nutritional therapy (MNT)

This is the mainstay of gestational diabetes treatment. Women with fasting blood glucose levels <95 mg/dL qualify for the trial of MNT; however, patients who are unable to achieve the target glycemic levels after 2 weeks may then need to initiate a pharmacologic therapy.

The Registered Dietitian should initiate Medical Nutrition Therapy within 1 week after diagnosis of GDM, and include at least three nutrition visits. Research indicates that early diagnosis of GDM and timely initiation of MNT results in improved

89

maternal and neonatal outcomes. Women suffering from GDM should receive nutritional counseling as well.

According to ADA nutrition practice guidelines, the clinical goals for treatment are to:

-Achieve and maintain euglycemia

-Consume adequate energy that promotes appropriate gestational weight gain and avoids maternal ketosis

-Consume food that provides nutrients essential for maternal and fetal health

A diet with less fat intake and a substitution of complex carbohydrates for refined carbohydrates helps to achieve and maintain an appropriate maternal blood glucose profile throughout gestation. The **ADA** recommends the patient to consult a registered dietitian to individualize a nutrition plan. The primary goal in MNT is to achieve euglycemia and also provide the required nutrients for fetal growth and proper maternal health; whereas, a secondary goal is to prevent excessive weight gain during pregnancy. Exercise potentially decreases peripheral insulin resistance and is a suitable adjunctive therapy to diet for the patient with GDM.

2) Nutrition Guidelines

-Focus on several dietary elements like calories, macronutrient proportion, vitamins and minerals, while considering age, physical activity and also stage of pregnancy.

-Approx. 30-40 Kcal/kg ideal body weight or an increment of 300kcal/day above the basal requirement is needed during 2nd and 3rd trimesters.

-Certain foods must be avoided in pregnancy due to fetal developmental harm, such as; smoked fish, unpasteurized milk, raw meat & eggs and also soft cheese. This is because of their association with bacterial infections. Fish containing mercury and raw shellfish should also be avoided.

Caffeine has been found to be associated with:

- Miscarriage

- Premature birth

- Low birth weight

- Withdrawal symptoms in the neonate (if consumed in larger amounts during pregnancy)

Avoid alcohol.

As a part of the MNT, it is advised to wisely distribute the calorie consumption throughout the day; especially breakfast. This involves splitting the usual breakfast portion into equal halves and then consuming them with a 2 hrs. gap in between. This avoids the undue peak in plasma glucose levels after ingestion of the complete breakfast.

3) The Fat content

The fat content in the American Diabetic Association diet consists of <25% of the total caloric intake. The saturated fatty acid has the ability to release better insulin during pregnancy.

The recommended dietary fat intake is to get 30-40% of calories from fat. Intake of cholesterol, saturated & trans fatty acids should be limited, whereas, intake of EPA (eicosapentaenoic acid; helps to reduce inflammation and blood clotting, dilates the blood vessels) and DHA (doceosahexaenoic acid; structural component in CNS) should be adequate (300 mg/day).

4) The Protein content

The protein content in the ADA euglycemic diet makes up 20% of the total daily caloric intake. Protein enriched meals increases satiety and therefore it could help morbidly obese patients to manage their overall caloric intake.

For the first trimester - 46g/day or .8g protein/kg/day

For the second and third trimester - 25g/day or 1.1g protein/kg

The maternal protein synthesis actually increases in order to support the expansion of the blood volume, uterus, and also the breasts.

5) Carbohydrate Intake

Although the ideal amount is unknown, it should be somewhere around 40-45% of the total daily energy intake. The recommended daily intake is 175g for pregnant women distributed throughout the day into 3 moderate sized meals and 2-4 snacks.

Folate requirement during pregnancy is 600µg/day. Deficiency may result in:

-Neural tube defect

-Down's syndrome

-Preterm delivery

-Elevated serum homocysteine level

An additional Iron intake (approx. 3mg/day) is required during pregnancy. An iron supplement of 30mg ferrous sulphate is recommended in the 2nd & 3rd trimesters (women are screened for iron status prior to pregnancy).

6) Pharmacologic Treatment Modalities for GDM

Pharmacotherapy is considered on the basis of monitoring maternal blood glucose with/without assessment of fetal growth characteristics. In cases where the optimal blood glucose levels have not been maintained with medical nutrition therapy (MNT) and/or the rate of fetal growth is excessive, the initiation of pharmacological therapy is then recommended for treatment of GDM. Research shows that pharmacological therapy, such as insulin and its analogs and oral medications improve glycemic control, thereby reducing the incidence of poor maternal and neonatal health outcomes.

a) Insulin therapy

Insulin is the only medication that is approved by FDA for the treatment of GDM. Insulin therapy is recommended by ADA when there are signs of either excessive fetal growth or poorly maintained maternal glycemic goals. It is safe and effective and is said to be the gold standard to which other therapies for GDM are compared. The safety profile of long-acting insulin during pregnancy has not been proven. The insulin treatment for GDM can be done in an outpatient clinic. The dosage of insulin is based on maternal weight, where according to one insulin regimen, the dose of insulin is calculated as 0.7 units/kg actual body weight. As seen, this dosage is lower compared to pregnant, non-GDM diabetic patients. This is a more conservative therapy, which is intended to prevent the hypoglycemia.

b) Dosing of Insulin

An insulin dose is always individualized and must be adjusted according to the needs of the patient. After calculating the total daily dosage, 2/3 of the dosage is administered before breakfast and the remaining 1/3 is broken up into 2 different doses.

The dose schedule of insulin requires modification depending upon the patent's BMI, glucose levels and also the lifestyle.

c) Insulin analogue

If the postprandial glucose remains uncontrolled, rapid acting insulin analogue is then considered. These have been found to be both safe and effective during pregnancy. A high dose of insulin may be required during pregnancy in pre-gestational diabetic women. A few of them may require multiple injections daily.

d) Oral Anti-diabetic Agents

Oral hypoglycemic agents can be used to control blood glucose when nutritional therapy has failed. The use of oral hypoglycemic medications in patients with GDM is contentious.

Glyburide is not FDA approved for treating GDM; however, there is supporting evidence that it can be used in conjunction with MNT and exercise for synergistic effects. It is the only sulfonylurea that has shown minimal placenta transfer and also shares no association with an excess neonatal hypoglycemia. One of the recent meta-analyses looked at three clinical trials that compared glyburide and insulin to find no statistically significant differences in the:

- Maternal outcomes

- Glycemic control

- Cesarean deliveries

- Neonatal outcomes

- Neonatal hypoglycemia

- Infant birth weight

The use of glyburide takes its origin from a study, *"A Comparison of Glyburide and Insulin in Women with Gestational Diabetes Mellitus"* where the researchers compared the efficacy and safety of glyburide versus insulin and reached a conclusion that the levels of glycemia, number of babies with macrosomia, neonatal hypoglycemia, and admission to neonatal intensive care units and fetal anomalies were equal in both research groups. With that, the incidence of maternal hypoglycemia was lower in the glyburide group compared to the insulin group.

Metformin is used off-label to treat GDM. It reduces insulin resistance by:

-Increasing the insulin sensitivity

-Reduces basal plasma insulin levels

-Stabilizes or facilitates weight reduction.

Moreover, metformin does not stimulate insulin secretion, which would otherwise subsequently cause hypoglycemia. The safety and efficacy of metformin in GDM has been examined by several clinical trials. Most of the researchers concluded through trials that metformin is safe and effective for GDM in the short-term.

Metformin can cross the placenta but any resultant fetal metabolic or teratogenic effects are unknown. In a research study conducted in 2008, the researchers concluded that metformin alone or with supplemental insulin is safe and effective to treat women with

GDM. More studies are required before recommending it for routine use during pregnancy.

First generation Sulphonyl ureas: (Tolbutamide and chlorpropamide) crosses the placenta and

can cause fetal hyperinsulinemia, leading to fetal macrosomia .

It can result in:

- prolonged neonatal hypoglycemia

- Profound and prolonged hyperinsulinemic (leading to fetal hypoxemia as a cause of late fetal death)

- Congenital malformations: first trimester sulfonylurea therapy associated with major congenital malformations but women with poorest metabolic control received sulfonylureas. Poor metabolic control is associated with congenital malformations.

Alpha-glucosidase Inhibitors (Acarbose): The use of Acarbose in pregnancy seems to be a good option because it primarily acts in the gut by delaying carbohydrate absorption and is not absorbed, thereby having no systemic effects. It is not systemically absorbed to an appreciable extent; therefore, trans-placental passage is not an issue. It is directly beneficial to the mother and indirectly to the fetus.

Women with GDM and treated with Acarbose have good glycemic control during the prenatal period. It prevents both maternal and fetal morbidity due to hyperglycemia. This medication appears to hold promise for the treatment of GDM, however, more studies are required before routinely recommending Acarbose in the management of gestational diabetes.

Chapter 11 : Emotional Health during Pregnancy with GDM

Stress is very common in today's lifestyle and is not good for your health. Unfortunately, it has more negative effects for people with diabetes. Either due to physical injury or some mental stress, it increases your heart rate and your blood pressure that might result in serious heart diseases. Stress can interfere with your sleep, causes sexual problems, stimulates appetite and triggers depression, anxiety and fatigue. This will collectively affect diabetes management. Chronic stress can even disturb the immune system of your body and can cause bone damage too. In general, in people with Diabetes Mellitus, stress, disturbed psychological state and depression have a direct effect on blood sugar levels.

1) How does stress affect blood sugar levels?
When an individual experiences stress, the body takes it as if it is being attacked and it needs to come into action either to face the situation or escape. It is called "fight or flight" condition. During this state, muscle tension, heart rate, breathing rate, blood pressure and blood flow to all parts of the body is increased. In addition, stress hormones e.g., *adrenaline* and *cortisol* are released to enhance the body's energy level by increasing the blood sugar level.

In normal individuals, the body recognizes this increase in the blood sugar levels and the pancreas responds to this by secreting more insulin. Insulin moves the sugar into the cells where it is used as energy. In diabetic patients, either insulin is lacking (Type

97

1 DM), or is not in sufficient amounts to fulfill the body's needs (Type 2 DM) in stressful conditions. That is why the blood sugar levels remain high during the fight-or-flight scenario. Another reason for high blood sugar levels could be the suppression of the pancreas' ability to secrete insulin due to increased stress hormones. It will further lessen the power or ability of the body to control blood glucose levels and to respond to stress.

2) Relaxation techniques can lower blood sugar levels and stress

Naturally, our body has an in-built mechanism for turning off the fight-or-flight response. It is known as the relaxation response of the body and it reverses all the physiological changes caused by stress. Stress response is usually imposed unwillingly so people can learn relaxation response intentionally as heart rate, breathing rate, muscle tension, glucose metabolism and blood pressure with blood sugar levels all decrease in relaxation response.

3) Relaxation techniques

The relaxation technique is the process that decreases stress on body and mind and helps you to cope with everyday stress and stress related to different health problems. Additionally, relaxation techniques also reduce labor pains and a number of unnecessary cesarean sections and enhance milk volume for lactating mothers.

4) Benefits of Relaxation techniques

Relaxation techniques help you to cope with various responsibilities of daily life including the demands of illness. Relaxation techniques reduce stress by:

-Slowing the heart rate

-Lowering B.P

-Increasing blood flow to major muscles

-Reducing muscle tension & pain

-Slowing the breathing rate

-Reducing frustration

-Improving concentration

-Enhancing confidence

Types of Relaxation Techniques that can be used in stress management are:

Autogenic Relaxation: This means something that comes from inside you. Both visual imagery and body awareness methods are used to reduce stress. In this, suggestions or words in your mind are repeated to reduce muscle tension and relax yourself. For example, focus on controlled breathing to slow your heart rate.

a) Deep breathing
Deeper and slower breathing is the antidote for stress and mental tension; it is also known as abdominal breathing. Anxiety and stress are counter balanced through this, as the blood pressure goes down and heart rate slows. One way to practice deep breathing is to lie on your back and place your hands over your chest and abdomen as you breathe. You should take in more air during this time and subsequently relax both muscles and mind.

b) Visualization
Mental images are formed to visualize peaceful and calming situations. You can use all your senses in this technique. For example, if you imagine yourself relaxing at the beach, think about the sound of crashing waves, the smell of salt water and the warmth of the sun etc. It could be used in pregnancy during labor,

as you may visualize yourself pushing baby out of the body with force and strength.

c) Progressive muscle relaxation
Each muscle group of the body is slowly tensed and then relaxed in this technique. It will help you to focus on the difference between muscle relaxation and tension. Tense your muscles for at least 5 seconds and then relax them for 30 seconds and repeat it for all the muscles of your body one by one starting from the head and neck down to your toes.

d) Other common relaxation techniques
*Massage

*Tai chi

*Yoga

*Hypnosis

*Meditation

*Aromatherapy

*Acupuncture

*Acupressure

*Mindfulness

*Yoga

*Biofeedback

e) Meditation
This is used to relax your mind and is done by concentrating your attention on the exercise that you are doing. Breathe normally

through your nose and prevent troubling thoughts from entering your mind. When you are in a relaxed meditative state, your blood pressure, blood sugar level and heart rate drops to normal, which makes your body fresh and stress-free.

f) Mindfulness
It involves moment-to-moment awareness i.e., focus only on the present task and don't let your mind wander to the worries.

g) Prenatal Yoga
This is another relaxing technique to deal with pregnancy stress. Yoga connects your mind with your body to minimize the tension and stress. It also improves balance and strengthens the body, which ultimately helps the pregnant woman to cope with changes in the body.

h) Touch therapies
Touch therapies are also very important in relaxing. Studies have shown that gentle touch on people with mental stress has a positive effect in reducing stress, depression and anxiety and increases relaxation and stamina of the body to cope with the situation.

i) Acupressure & Acupuncture
Acupuncture is the insertion of sterilized needles into the skin at specific pressure points in the body. In Acupressure, fingers are used to apply manual pressure at particular acupoints on the body. These Acupoints are used to restore the body's balance and health. They are used to control nausea and vomiting related to pregnancy.

Pain in the lower back and pelvic area is most common in later months due to weight gain. Acupuncture and Acupressure are effective in pain relief and management without any medicine.

j) Biofeedback

This trains the patient to control the blood flow, heart rate and muscle tension throughout the body in order to reach a state of deep relaxation. It will result in reduced blood pressure, reduced stress hormone levels and pain. It can even diminish the effects of certain heart diseases as well.

k) Hypnosis

The success of hypnosis therapy on diabetics depends on following three factors:

The patient's motivation and ability to establish rapport with the doctor, the patient's trust of the physician's skill and his ability to hypnotize them and the understanding of the patient about hypnosis (that it will lead to a positive change).

These exercises can help you to focus your attention inwards as your body will receive a message that you are secure and your muscles will relax as a result of the reduction in stress. Your pulse rate will drop and your anxiety will decrease. Before starting the practice, make sure that conditions are suitable for you, for example:

Privacy: Avoid places where you can be disturbed. Pick a quiet place and close the door.

Comfort: Sit on a comfortable chair and close your eyes.

Concentration: Concentrate on what you are doing, if your thoughts wander, refocus your attention.

Duration: Practice at least 10 minutes every day. Once you have relaxed, your efficiency will improve and you can work more effectively.

5) Dealing with Diabetes related stress

Some stresses of life never go away, no matter what you do. Having diabetes is one of those. Certain periods of life can be more difficult than others with diabetes. For example, *when you are diagnosed* you will feel physically unwell. To know about the fact that you have a chronic disease can result in deep feelings of grief and loss. Or you may feel anxious when first diagnosed as you may know someone who is suffering with diabetes. Their experience may color your thinking. This can cause a further sense of fear, pressure or anxiety.

6) When you experience a life transition

To deal with diabetes when you are making changes in your life can be more difficult as going through transitions often takes up a lot of energy. It can result in less energy left to manage the diabetes. When diabetes interferes with life's priorities, feeling of anger and frustration become more severe. The use of Insulin could be the big change in many people's life as they need to monitor it regularly and more attention to the timings of meals and exercise patterns is required.

7) If you develop complications of Diabetes

Significant readjustments are required if you develop any complications of diabetes. If it affects your vision then you may need to concentrate harder on tasks requiring alertness. If it makes you less mobile, you may feel that you are dependent on others. Depending on the severity of the complications, you may feel great grief associated with the loss of full health. Having diabetes is stressful and it makes it difficult to manage other life stresses also. As you experience more with diabetes, you become used to it and you achieve a comfortable balance between caring for yourself and enjoying your life. Stress management strategies become more effective at that time.

The effects of stress in people with type 1 diabetes mellitus are random, while most people's blood glucose levels go high with mental stress and other's blood glucose levels can go down. In type 2 diabetes, mental stress raises blood sugar levels. Physical stress results in higher blood sugar levels in people with either type of DM. For diabetic people, controlling stress with relaxation therapy seems to be helpful. But it is more effective in people with type 2 diabetes than people with type 1 diabetes. It might be because stress blocks the release of insulin in the body of someo,e with type 2 diabetes, so reducing stress may be more helpful in these patients. People with type 1 diabetes don't produce insulin so stress cutting doesn't affect it. People with type 2 diabetes are more sensitive to stress hormones also and relaxing can help by reducing this sensitivity.

Other *ways to reduce the stresses* of living with diabetes are support groups. Knowing other people with the same condition may help you feel less alone. You can learn important tips from other people for coping with problems. Making friends can also help in lightening the burden of diabetes-related stress. Dealing directly with diabetes care issues can also help to reduce stress. Counseling or psychotherapy can be done to reduce stresses and talking with a therapist may help you to find out ways to deal with your problems. You may learn new ways of changing your behavior or new ways of coping.

8) Pregnancy and Stress

Although pregnancy is considered as a time of great joy, it's not the same for all women and one in ten pregnant women suffers from depression. Pregnancy brings out worry in women for a good reason as you are growing a life inside of you. So it is natural to worry about what you feel, eat, drink, think and do. It is normal to worry about the baby's health also as this new person will change your life and relationships.

Experts believe that at the start of pregnancy, there is a rapid increase in hormone levels that can disrupt brain chemistry and lead to depression. Hormonal changes can make you feel more anxious than usual but if your anxiety is regularly interfering with your daily tasks then it's the time to find a better way to deal with this anxiety. Anxiety and depression may go undiagnosed because women don't share their feelings but it is advised not to feel shy about sharing it with your doctor if you feel low. Emotional health is just as important as your physical health, in fact, it can affect your physical health as well. For example, depression and anxiety can increase the risk of preterm labor.

9) Common Pregnancy Stresses

A stress-free pregnancy is not possible and when you accept this fact make sure that you know how to deal with the stress. The common stresses that you may experience during pregnancy could be the same as you may experience any other time (money or work etc) with the additional stress of taking care of yourself and to preparing yourself for the time when the baby comes. Before dealing with the stress, the most important thing is to find out the reason behind that stress so that you can do something to eliminate it from your life. If it cannot be eliminated then try to develop some plan to handle it with less stress. For example, if your stress is financial, create a budget and plan to stick to it.

10) Healthy ways to handle Pregnancy Stress:

If you are worried and stressed, try different things that can help you to feel better and that keep you away from its bad effects on your health and pregnancy.

11) The following things can be used to deal with your stress:

Talk it out: Find a person that you can trust and with whom you can share your problem. Make sure that this person helps to keep you positive.

Try breathing exercises and meditation: Breathing deeply in a quiet, separated environment can help you to get rid of your stress.

Get plenty of rest: Rest is important for everyone, but it becomes more important when your body works more during the gestation period to take care of you and the fetus inside you.

Try prenatal yoga: It is a good way to exercise during gestation as Yoga promotes clarity and relaxation and helps in dealing with stresses.

Pamper yourself: Having a newborn child will certainly cut down your time for yourself, however taking time for yourself is the best way to relieve stress. So, stock up before the baby arrives and take lots of opportunities for massages, bubble baths, manicures and pedicures.

One or more of these tools can be used to deal with your stress and the more you use these techniques, the better you are, which in turn will result in better effects to your unborn baby.

12) Common Risk Factors:
- Problems with your pregnancy
- Personal or family history of depression
- Previous pregnancy loss

- Relationship difficulties
- Past history of abuse
- Fertility treatments
- Stressful events
- Other risk factors including unplanned pregnancy

13) Symptoms of Depression

Common symptoms of stress among healthy women during pregnancy are fatigue or trouble sleeping. But when these symptoms are combined with sad feelings or hopelessness, they may interfere with your ability to function.

Talk to your healthcare provider about what you feel if you experience three or more of the following *symptoms*:

- Trouble sleeping or sleeping all the time
- Difficulty concentrating
- A sense that nothing feels fun anymore
- Feeling sad or "empty" most days
- Never ending fatigue
- Extreme irritability or excessive crying
- Severe agitation
- Feelings of hopelessness
- Desire to eat all the time or not wanting to eat at all.
- Mood swings with cycles of depression, combined with periods of abnormally high spirits are the signs of a serious condition called "bipolar disorder" and it requires immediate attention.

Consult your caregiver if you have the following symptoms:

-Inappropriate social behavior
-Increased activity
-Racing thoughts

-Little or no sleep

-Little or no eating

-Poor judgment

14) Symptoms of Anxiety

Call your doctor or midwives if you are feeling any of the following symptoms:

- Frequent and recurrent concerns about your health or about your baby's health
- Frequently feeling like something terrible is about to happen
- Panic attacks including a racing heart and sweaty palms, lightheadedness, breathlessness, faintness or feelings of having a heart attack.

Stress, depression and anxiety all are not good for your health and may result in serious health consequences either for you or for your baby.

Your level of stress will directly affect your fetus's health. Everyone in today's lifestyle faces some sort of pressure in their daily life but high levels of chronic stress can enhance the possibility of mishaps such as preterm labor or low-birth weight delivery. If you are used to stress in your routine life, due to your work load or any other kind of stress, making yourself priority may seem selfish or unnatural. But during pregnancy, taking care of yourself is an essential part of taking care of your baby. So learn to cut down stress and learn how to manage your work load with less stress and make your pregnancy healthier.

15) How are anxiety and depression treated during pregnancy?

The elaxation techniques mentioned above can be used to treat stress and depression according to the advice of your healthcare professional. Other than that, antidepressants and psychotherapy can be used to treat these conditions during gestation. Hozever, don't try to self-medicate yourself and don't try St. John's Wort or any other remedy without consulting your doctor. This is for your own health and safety as the safety of these remedies during pregnancy is unknown and they are not an effective substitute for professional help.

16) What to do with postpartum depression

Postpartum anxiety and depression are very common among women who suffer from depression during gestation period. But if they were treated during pregnancy then it can reduce the chances of developing postpartum depression. Here are few things to do:

-Divide your household responsibilities after talking with your partner and take care of each other as well as your baby.

-Make a habit of taking care of yourself as it becomes part of your routine. Plan different ways to get some time off to rest once the baby come.

-Join a support network

-Learn to manage your household responsibilities in such a way that you can grab some time for baby care and for own self.

Chapter 12 : Life After Gestational Diabetes

Life after gestational diabetes will never be normal as women may suffer from any of the postpartum issues related to Gestational Diabetes. Women who had gestational diabetes are at a high risk of developing GDM in subsequent pregnancies and type 2 diabetes later in life.

In most cases, blood glucose levels will return to normal after delivery, but according to studies, the reoccurrence rate of GDM ranges from 30% to 65%. Women with GDM are at risk of developing type 2 diabetes with a ratio of 40% to 60%.

1) Postpartum risk factors for developing diabetes:

* Degree of abnormality of glucose tolerance test

* Family history of type 2 diabetes

* Degree of obesity

* Certain ethnicities

* Pre-pregnancy weight

* Age

* Degree of hyperglycemia in pregnancy and after delivery.

2) Strategies in Postpartum care

* Changes in lifestyle habits

* Counseling to promote healthy food

* Weight management

* Regular physical activities.

3) Postpartum screening and diagnosis

Postpartum screening for all the women with GDM is important as it helps to identify women who are likely to have diabetes. It should be done 6 to 12 weeks after delivery according to the recommendations of the American Diabetes Association to ensure normal blood glucose levels. Women with a history of GDM should be tested for reassessment of blood glycemic levels every 3 years. Women with impaired glucose tolerance should be tested annually. There is a 50% chance of developing type 2 diabetes within 5 years if you have had a history of GDM.

4) Manage your weight gain (for post-partum obesity sufferers)

Weight management is very important for women with a history of GDM as with increased weight the chances of getting diabetes becomes stronger. Insulin resistance is triggered as fat accumulates in the body in overweight people. Being overweight may also lead to high blood pressure and heart disease. Studies have shown that weight loss reduces the insulin resistance associated with decreased blood sugar in people with type 2 diabetes. Weight loss also results in decreased blood triglyceride levels, blood cholesterol and blood pressure. Furthermore, weight loss works effectively against several other diseases.

5) Postpartum weight management with physical activity

Weight management is possible with some regular physical activity and exercise. Pregnancy has been considered as a diabetogenic event as hormones lead to increased insulin requirements and insulin resistance. It results in low blood glucose levels and to compensate an increase in insulin secretions

111

occurs throughout the gestation period. Patients with GDM have decreased insulin sensitivity due to increased fat storage. This impaired insulin sensitivity results in decreased glucose uptake by organs and muscles, with increased hepatic glucose production. Exercise has been reported as an adjunctive method in GDM management as during exercise catecholamine are released to stimulate gluconeogenesis.

Pregnancy induces anxiety and stress in women, and if GDM is also diagnosed then it will put a greater load on a woman, physically and emotionally. Regular exercising is one easy way that can help prevent a high risk of GDM and to manage it in a better way. It will also help high risk women to avoid the onset of type 2 diabetes later in life.There is a strong relationship between increased weight loss and enhanced exercise activities in the first year after delivery. Women having any complications should consult their doctor to know which exercises are suitable for her.

Physical activity including exercise is strongly recommended to GDM patients as it will lower blood glucose levels and will also help to regain pre-pregnancy weight. Furthermore, exercise is more acceptable and less stressful than insulin injections for women. The most frequently and easily adapted physical activity for maintaining weight gain is walking. Other possible options are yoga, aerobic activities and swimming.

6) The benefits of postpartum physical activity

There are so many benefits of physical activities in the postpartum period. It helps in weight loss, decreases urinary stress incontinence, increases energy and moods and has the following effects:

- Less depression and anxiety

- More relaxed relationship between child and mother

- Improved bladder control

- Improved perception of new relationship between mother and child

- Less lactation-induced loss of bone mass

- Less pregnancy-induced weight retention.

7) Exercises to Avoid in postpartum period

Hormonal changes occur during pregnancy and cause ligamentous and core instability. It might continue in the postpartum period also and may extend until the new mother is lactating the new born. Because of this reason, women may need to avoid some specific exercises including thigh adduction, squats, and lunges; they must be avoided for at least 6 weeks after delivery until the doctor clears the new mother. The duration to avoid these exercises may extend depending upon the nursing status of the mother and on the core and pelvic strength.

8) Barriers to physical activity

Possible barriers to physical activities in the post-partum period may include:

- Lack of time

- Lack of child care

- Lack of enjoyment of physical activity

- Feeling tired

- Unsuitable local neighborhood.

- Lack of knowledge about the importance of physical activity in managing weight gain & diabetes prevention postpartum in GDM patients.

9) How Can I Avoid Future Risks?

Studies have shown that about 60% of women with a history of GDM develop type 2 DM within 5-15 years after pregnancy. Factors affecting impaired glucose tolerance in type 2 DM includes age of mother, glycemic levels in pregnancy & postpartum during OGTT, obesity and diagnosis of GDM before 24 week's pregnancy. The risk of developing GDM in subsequent pregnancies is 30% to 65% in women with a history of GDM. Predictors for developing DM in high risk women are Preterm delivery and elevated fasting glycemic levels.

Factors that increase the risk of recurrence of GDM include:

-Hip to waist ratio

-Diet composition

-Weight gained during pregnancies. Studies have shown that a woman with a history of GDM is at twice the risk of developing diabetes or impaired glucose intolerance during 4-8 years after pregnancy than control subjects without any history of GDM.

Cardiovascular Disease Risks:

There is a relation between cardiovascular risk factors and impaired fasting glucose and impaired glucose tolerance in women with a history of GDM. Impaired glucose metabolism is associated with cardiovascular risks as there is an increased incidence of higher diastolic blood pressure and triglycerides in women with impaired glucose tolerance and impaired fasting glucose than in women with normal blood glucose levels.

The National Cholesterol Education Program's Adult Treatment Plan III (ATP III) shifts the focus from dietary steps to "therapeutic lifestyle changes" (TLC) reinforcing the combined importance of dietary intake and physical activities in weight management to reduce the incidence of heart diseases and to avoid the development of diabetes.

10) Long term diabetes risk

Women with GDM should be informed about the risks of developing type 2 DM. Primary preventive healthcare for all women with or without diabetes is the main priority for all the healthcare providers.

Prevention of type 2 DM in high risk women with a history of GDM can be done by the following strategies:

- Education about risk awareness

- Implementation of healthy life style

- Changing eating habits

- Breast-feeding

- Pharmacotherapy.

11) Risk Awareness

Although gestational diabetes mellitus is a well-established risk factor for type 2 diabetes mellitus, many women with GDM are unaware of this risk. It could be one of the reasons of reduced compliance with the recommendation to avoid the risk of diabetes. One of the studies conducted about risk awareness has shown that 47% of women with GDM history believe that it was "highly possible" to develop type 2 DM, whereas 35% believe that it was "somewhat" possible. Another study revealed that 90%

115

of women with GDM history were aware of future risks of developing DM. But there was a group of women who didn' believe that GDM has any risks after pregnancy in later life.

It is concluded that interventions are required to increase the awareness and acceptance of the risks for development of type 2 diabetes in women with a GDM history at an individual level. Public education campaigns could help in increasing risk awareness in patients. Centers for disease control and prevention, and different conferences and online information are other ways to increase the awareness of health risks for women with GDM history.

12) Postpartum counseling

Postpartum counseling is equally important as are other interventions in women with a GDM history to avoid the risk of the recurrence of GDM in subsequent pregnancies and of type 2 diabetes later in life. After delivery all women should be tested to screen and diagnose DM by either fasting plasma glucose level or 2-hour oral glucose tolerance test. The frequency of testing is not established so it depends on the caregiver and according to the severity of risk factors, if any are present e.g., obesity, ethnicity and early gestational age at diagnosis and fasting hyperglycemia during pregnancy. Importantly, women with a DM history should be screened before planning the subsequent pregnancy. Furthermore, women should be encouraged to adopt healthy lifestyle modifications to decrease insulin resistance. Regular walking should be encouraged to maintain weight and to avoid weight gain and obesity. Insulin-sensitizing drug therapy helps in delaying or preventing the development of diabetes by reducing insulin resistance in high-risk women with history of GDM.

13) Lifestyle modification

Another intervention to control the risks of developing type 2 diabetes in women with history of GDM is lifestyle modification. The ACOG and the ADA both recommend that women with a history of GDM are at risk of developing diabetes, and that they should be counseled about the combined benefits of diet, exercise and weight loss in obese women in order to prevent the development of diabetes. Studies demonstrate that intensive lifestyle modification can reduce the incidence of type 2 diabetes in people with impaired glucose tolerance. There is a need to carry out studies to evaluate the most effective way to achieve lifestyle modification in people with a history of GDM.

14) Breast-feeding

Breast-feeding is one of the effective means to reduce blood glucose levels. It is suggested to high risk women with history of GDM to continue breast-feeding after delivery. It will also help in reducing the incidence of Type 2 Diabetes Mellitus in women with a history of GDM and in the general population also. Lactation is also associated with low prevalence of metabolic syndrome and postpartum reduced long-term obesity risk and weight loss. Studies have shown that there is an inverse relation between type 2 Diabetes Mellitus and the duration of breast-feeding. Breast-feeding within the first 12 hours helps to stimulate the onset of Lactogenesis in women with type 1 DM.

Biochemical markers for lactation including sodium, lactose, citrate and total proteins and the milk volume both appear to be delayed in type 1 diabetic woman for about 24 hours. But the quality of breast-milk is not affected in diabetic women with good health and good metabolic control. Lower diabetes rates and lower maternal blood glucose levels are observed in breast-feeding women with GDM during postpartum period.

Weight-loss benefits:

Lactation will help in losing weight in women with GDM in the postpartum period if energy intake is not increased. The estimated milk energy output is approximately 500kcal/day in the first 6 months and 400kcal/day in the second 6 months of breast-feeding.

a) Effects on Glucose Metabolism

As glucose is required in breast-milk synthesis, it could be the possible reason of lowering maternal blood glucose levels. The only carbohydrate found in milk is lactose and glucose is required for its synthesis and volume of milk produced. The estimated concentration of lactose in breast-milk is 72g/ L. Lactose synthesis increases glucose utilization by 30% more in lactating mothers.

Different studies are performed to find the relation between blood glucose concentrations and breast-feeding in type 1 DM mothers, and it is found that lactating women have shown improved glucose tolerance. Insulin requirements are also decreased in the postpartum period of GDM with type 1 DM in lactating mothers compared to non-lactating mothers.

b) Daily nutritional requirements

The nutritional needs of lactating women with a history of GDM in pregnancy are the same as the nutritional requirements of lactating women without a GDM history.

c) Nutritional advice for lactation after GDM in the postpartum period

- Choose a variety of food everyday

- Have 3 meals or snacks/day

- Drink to satisfy thirst and don't take excessive fluids

118

- Have 3 or more servings of milk items

- Take multivitamin supplements with iron regularly

- Limit tea or coffee to 1 cup/day

- Limit the use of non-nutritive sweeteners.

d) The effect of nutrition on the composition of milk

A woman's prenatal nutrition, nutrient intake during pregnancy, amount of weight gained during pregnancy, and changes in her eating habits including disease related adaptation, dieting and supplements intake can all affect human milk composition.

The following recommendations from the Institute of Medicine can help to understand the relation between nutrition and milk composition:

-A diet with less than 1500kcal/day can decrease the milk volume in lactating mothers

-The amount of saturated and unsaturated fatty acids in a diet will affect their concentration in the milk

-Vitamin concentration in breast-milk is dependent on maternal stores and food intake.

-Calcium and Folate concentration in breast-milk is maintained at the expense of maternal stores

-Diet intake has no effect on phospholipid and cholesterol concentration in human milk.

e) Breast-feeding and Exercises

Some people might think that exercising in the postpartum period in women with GDM to lose weight will affect milk production quantitatively or qualitatively but it's not true. Exercise doesn't decrease milk production but it does increase the amount of lactic acid in breast-milk. Exercising doesn't affect the infant's weight gain or length trajectory. If an infant rejects post-exercise then collect milk pre-exercise and pump and discard post-exercise milk.

Studies have shown that the combination of physical activity, proper diet and lactation after pregnancy with GDM can eliminate the risk of diabetes in mothers without affecting infant growth.

Guidelines for exercise and breast-feeding include:

- Choose mild to moderate exercise

- Avoid exhaustive & strenuous exercise

- Exercise after baby is fed

- Wear a good support bra and avoid breast compression

- Ensure adequate hydration before, during and after the physical activity

- Take Vitamin B6 and Calcium supplements if daily intake is not adequate

- Ensure sufficient caloric intake that supports both exercise and lactation.

Chapter 13: Obesity

There is strong evidence that weight gain, obesity and physical inactivity are the main risk factors that may lead to the development of type 2 diabetes. Abdominal obesity is the important cause in the pathogenesis of insulin resistance. Free fatty acids produced by the adipocyte impair glucose utilization by the skeletal muscles, promotes gluconeogenesis by the liver, and may impair β-cell function directly. Each of these factors play an important role in insulin resistance development.

Hypertensive disease of pregnancy occurs with the frequency 2-4 times in obese mothers. The association between raised BMI and pre-eclamptic toxemia (PET) occurs in women with GDM and glucose tolerant mothers. Other complications such as pelvic pain and lower back pain are more common in overweight and obese mothers during gestation. Maternal obesity is also associated with a higher rate of labor induction, which requires higher prostaglandins and higher oxytocin compared to women with a normal BMI.

Maternal obesity is one of the major risk factors for maternal mortality. Obesity related mishaps can extend into the postpartum period and beyond. Adverse outcomes of obesity cannot be explained by its contribution in maternal hyperglycemia and/or development of GDM. Adverse outcomes of obesity also contribute in glucose tolerant women.

1) Fetal and neonatal outcome

Raised pre-pregnancy maternal BMI may result in the increased risk of macrosomia with highest risks for large for gestational age (LGA) birth weight. Possible immediate neonatal complications are also associated with maternal obesity including hypoglycemia, respiratory distress syndrome and hyperbilirubinemia.

2) Chronic Inflammation in obesity

In obese people, serum markers of inflammation are raised, whichis due to the activation of pro-inflammatory elements of the immune system. Studies have shown that the blood levels of pro-inflammatory cytokines such as interleukin (IL), IL-6, tumor necrosis factor (TNF), and monocytes chemo attractant proteins are increased during pregnancy. The chronic inflammatory process that is associated with obesity extends to the placenta during pregnancy that will lead to direct fetal adverse effects. Many of the adverse pregnancy outcomes are independently related to the obesity of the mother. Therefore, the relation between abnormal glucose balance, insulin resistance and chronic inflammation is well established.

3) Body weight and obesity

Body weight and obesity both affect the health of the mother and newborn and can increase the complications. So weight management in obese mothers is more important than in over-weight mothers. They should be encouraged during individualized counseling to reduce weight, decrease saturated fats and total fats intake and an increase in fiber intake. Studies have shown that obese mothers with impaired glucose tolerance can delay their progression to type 2 diabetes mellitus by losing weight.

Obesity triggers type 2 diabetes mellitus because of increase in visceral fat in those obese individuals. Central obesity is the major predictive of type 2 diabetes mellitus and it is measured indirectly by skin folds or waist-to-hip ratio. Insulin sensitivity improves with weight loss and it is increased to the greater extent with decreased waist-to-hip ratio and decreased abdominal fats.

After delivery, weight management in women with a history of GDM can be done by dietetics professionals. According to the *American Dietetic Association*, an assessment of a woman's weight and health status is important to determine the treatment plan.

The assessment consists of the following parameters:

Medical: Identifying potential causes, severity of obesity and associated disorders.

Psychological: Identifying the barriers to the treatment.

Anthropometric: Measuring BMI, current weight, height, and waist circumference.

Nutritional: Determine diet history, weight history, current eating pattern, nutrition intake, exercise history, environmental factors, women's motivation and readiness to change.

1) Management strategies for maternal obesity

Maternal obesity and weight reduction can be done by :

- Regular exercise

- Regular monitoring of glycemic levels

- Regular risk awareness counseling

- Educational programs or campaigns

- Lifestyle modification

- Regular healthy and low calories food intake

- Social support with family support

- Medications including Metformin

- Physical activities

- Medical nutrition therapy

2) Contraception

As we discussed, women who have had GDM have more chances of developing it again in subsequent pregnancies. It may further lead to the development of type 2 diabetes later in life or before the next pregnancy, making it difficult for mother and fetus too if it is not diagnosed or treated. For this reason, it is extremely important to prevent accidental pregnancies. If the blood glucose level is high at the time of conception, then the rate of miscarriages and birth defects is comparatively high. Blood glucose levels should be tested to be normal before next conception and you should follow a diabetic food plan before beginning to attempt to conceive.

In order to avoid accidental pregnancy when blood glucose levels are unknown, you must use very reliable form of birth control. Birth control has a significant failure rate in the first year after pregnancy, and you must take special care in using birth control.

3) The importance of planning pregnancy and the role of contraception

The importance of avoiding an unplanned pregnancy is the essential component of diabetes education for women with diabetes. Women who are planning on becoming pregnant should be advised that the risks associated with pregnancy get more complicated with diabetes and also increase with the duration of diabetes.

Other important points of educating women with diabetes are the use of contraceptive pills until good glycemic control is achieved, glucose monitoring, the glycemic targets, medications for diabetes and medications for treating complications associated with diabetes. These all need to be reviewed before, during and after pregnancy.

Additional effort and time is required to manage diabetes during pregnancy and frequent contact with healthcare professionals will be required for that. Women should be provided with information about emergency contact numbers and local arrangements for support

4) Contraception Methods & Birth Control Choices

Different ways are available to avoid unplanned pregnancy. Only you and your partner can decide what the right method is for you, among many available forms of birth control. Some types of birth control are not recommended for women with the history of GDM in pregnancy due to unavailability of insufficient data.

a) Barrier Methods

This includes diaphragms, condoms and cervical caps. They tend to be the best choice for post-partum birth control until breastfeeding has been continuing for quite some time. Condoms can be used without any problem. Changes in a woman's body makes other barrier methods less effective including cervical caps and diaphragms.

Advantages of Barrier methods:

- They don't affect blood lipids or blood glucose

- Unlike oral contraceptives and implants they don't interfere with the hormonal levels of your body

- They have no effect on breast milk and don't decrease supply, and don't affect the baby's natural system

- They will not increase the chances of developing diabetes later in life

Disadvantages of Barrier methods:

- Less spontaneous to use

- Higher user failure rate

Spontaneity can be treated by being more creative. In addition, the failure rate (due to using it incorrectly, inconsistently or in ignorance) can be significantly lower in people who are more responsible about birth control and protection.

b) Oral Contraceptives
This is a very popular form of birth control but should be used with caution to decide which type of pill should be used due to the facts that some pills can worsen blood lipids, bring on diabetes or interfere with breast-feeding supply. It is probably best to avoid all oral contraceptives if you have GDM and you are breast-feeding your new born.

Care must be taken in deciding which type of pill should be used. The new type of contraceptive pills are either low dose combination pills of estrogen and progestin or low dose "mini-pills" of progestin only. It is not sure whether these pills are safe to use for women with a history of GDM or not but it is extremely important to know that types and doses of contraceptive pills vary strongly and need to be researched before usage. It is important to take into account all possible risk factors like hypertension, smoking, age, breast-feeding etc. Frequent follow-ups are very important for women with gestational diabetes after beginning an oral contraceptive.

c) Implants/ Injections

These are not a good option for women with a history of GDM. Another factor is that the progesterone hormone in injections and implants come in high doses and can bring back the diabetes into your pre-pregnant state. So they are not the first-choice contraceptives for women with previous gestational diabetes.

d) Intra-Uterine Devices (IUDs)

This gives a long-acting and effective contraceptive that does not involve metabolic or hormonal disturbance. It has a low failure rate but it is contraindicated in some cases. Multiple sex partners, history of ectopic pregnancy, history of chronic pelvic infections, or history of sexually transmitted disease are the contraindications for use of UDIs. It prevents the implantation of a fertilized egg so some women may have moral/religious objections.

e) Surgical sterilization

Lastly, surgical sterilization is an excellent choice for women no longer having interest in childbearing. It is a good option as sterilization can be performed during the surgical procedure of cesarean section.

In *conclusion*, it is vital that women with a history of GDM have different options for birth control and generally can use all forms of contraception according to standard guidelines provided (mentioned above in the table). The only exception is progestin-only methods as they should be avoided or used with caution during lactation. Women with a history of GDM require safe and effective contraception that suits their lifestyle without enhancing the risk of developing metabolic syndrome, cardiovascular problems or diabetes mellitus. Regardless of the method used, care plans should be individualized. Regular screening of lipid disorders and surveillance of glucose tolerance and other cardiovascular risk factors should be carried out. A healthy lifestyle should be reinforced and blood pressure monitoring and weight management should be done regularly.

Further Studies
*Handbook of Diabetes:

A John Wiley & Sons, Ltd., Publication

Rudy Bilous MD, FRCP Professor of Clinical Medicine, Newcastle University

Honorary Consultant Endocrinologist, South Tees Foundation Trust, Middleborough, UK

Richard Donnelly MD, PHD, FRCP, FRACP Head, School of Graduate Entry Medicine and Health, University of Nottingham Honorary Consultant Physician, Derby Hospitals NHS Foundation Trust, Derby, UK 4th edition.

---

*American Dietetic Association Guide to Gestational Diabetes Mellitus by Alyce M. Thomas, Yolanda Monroy Gutierrez.

---

*Gestational Diabetes During and After Pregnancy

By Catherine Kim, Assiamira Ferrara

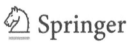 Springer
Springer. Copyright.

---

*Gestational Diabetes: New Insights for the Healthcare Professional:

2013 edition.

*Joslin's Diabetes Mellitus: Edited by C. Ronald Kahn ... [et Al.].

Edited by Elliott Proctor Joslin, C. Ronald Kahn

*The Treatment of Diabetes Mellitus with Chinese Medicine: A Textbook & Clinical Manual

By Bob Flaws, Lynn M. Kuchinski, Robert Casañas.

Textbook of Perinatal Medicine, Second Edition edited by Asim Kurjak, Frank A. Chervenak.

References

*Alexander, G., N. Sehgal, R. Moloney, and R. Stafford. 2008. National trends in treatment of type 2 diabetes mellitus, 1994–2007. Archives of Internal Medicine 168 (19): 2088–94.

*American Diabetes Association. 2008. All about diabetes. diabetes.org/about-diabetes.jsp. Anderson, J. E. 2006. A patient with type 2 diabetes and cirrhosis of the liver, Clinical Diabetes (24): 43–44.

*Anonymous. 1965. Diabetes: A scope monograph on the nature, diagnosis, and treatment of diabetes mellitus. Kalamazoo, MI: Upjohn Company. --Bennett, J. C. and F. Plum, eds. 1996. -Cecil textbook of medicine. 20th ed. Philadelphia: W. B. Saunders.

*Busse, F. P., P. Hiermanna, A. Gallera, M. Stumvollb, T. Wiessnerb, W. Kiessa, and T. Kapellena. 2007. Evaluation of patients' opinion and metabolic control after transfer of young adults with type 1 diabetes from a pediatric diabetes clinic to adult care. Hormone Research 67 (3): 132–38.

*Centers for Disease Control and Prevention, CDC. 2005. National diabetes fact sheet: General information and national estimates on diabetes in the United States. Atlanta, GA: U.S. Department of Health and Human Services.

*Ceriello, A., and S. Colagiuri. 2008. International Diabetes Federation guideline for management of post-meal glucose: A review of recommendations. Diabetic Medicine 25 (10): 1151–56.

*Crea, R., A. Kraszewski, T. Hirose, and K. Itakura. 1978. Chemical synthesis of genes for human insulin. Proceedings of the National Academy of Sciences 75 (12): 5765–69.

References

*Dean, L. 2004. -Introduction to diabetes. National Center for Biotechnology, Information website. ncbi.nlm.nih.gov/bookshelf/br.fcgi?book=diabetes&part=A5.Fow ler, M. J. 2008.Hypoglycemia. Clinical Diabetes 26:170–73.

*Frank, R. N. 2004.Diabetic retinopathy. New England Journal of Medicine 350 (1): 48–58.

*Harris, E. H. 2005. Elevated liver function tests in type 2 diabetes. Clinical Diabetes

23:115–19.

*Hilsted, J. 1982. Pathophysiology in diabetic autonomic neuropathy: Cardiovascular, hormonal, and metabolic studies. Diabetes 31:730–37.

*Imura, H. 2000. Diabetes: Current perspectives. New England Journal of Medicine 342:1533.

*Isselbacher, K., E. Braunwald, J. Wilson, J. Martin, A. Fauci, and D. Kasper, eds. 1994.Harrison's principles of internal medicine. 13th Ed. New York: McGraw-Hill.

*Lefebvre, P. 2002. Diabetes yesterday, today and tomorrow: Work of the International Federation of Diabetes. Bulletin ET Memoires de l'Academie Royale de Medecine de Bel-gique 157 (10–12): 455–63.

*Macleod, J. 1925. Insulin: Its use in the treatment of diabetes. Baltimore, MD: Williams and Wilkins.Marks, J. B. 2003. Clinical diabetes and the diabetes epidemic, Clinical Diabetes 21:2–3.MoveForward. 2009. The alarming statistics on diabetes. Diabetes Forum website: diabetesforum.com/blog/2009/06/the-alarming-statistics-on-diabetes.

References

*National Geographic Society. 1998. National Geographic eyewitness to the 20th century. Washington, DC: National Geographic Society.

*Peters, A. 2005. Conquering diabetes: A complete program for prevention and treatment, New York: Plume.

*Reaven, G. M. 1988. Banting lecture: Role of insulin resistance in human disease. Diabetes 37:1595–1607.

*Serri, O. 1991. Somatostatin analogue, octreotide, reduces increased glomerular filtra-tion rate and kidney size in insulin-dependent diabetes. Journal of the American Medi-cal Association 265 (7): 888–92.

*Shro, R. J. 2004. Case study: Screening and treatment of prediabetes in primary care. Clinical Diabetes 22:98–100.

*Smeltzer, S., and B. Bare. 2004. Medical-surgical nursing. Vol. 1. 10th ed. (Philippine). Philadelphia: Lippincott. Smeltzer, S., and B. Bare. 2004. Medical-surgical nursing. Vol. 2. 10th ed. (Philippine). Philadelphia: Lippincott.

*Stretton, A. 2002. The first sequence: Fred Sanger and insulin. Genetics 162 (2): 527–32.

*Ward, W., J. Beard, J. Halter, M. Pfeifer, and D. Porte Jr. 1984. Pathophysiology of insulin secretion in non-insulin-dependent diabetes mellitus, Diabetes Care 7:491–502.

*Williamson, R. T. 1898. Diabetes mellitus and its treatment, London: Pentland.

*Wilson, M. 2008. Carbohydrates, proteins, and fats, Merck website: merck.com/mmhe/sec12/ch152/ch152b.html.

133

*American Diabetes Association. 2004. Hyperglycemic crises in diabetes. Clinical practice recommendations, Diabetes Care 27 (Suppl. 1): S94–S102.References 221.

*American Diabetes Association. 2007. Type 2 Diabetes. Author website. www.diabetes.org/type-2-diabetes.jsp.

*Aronovitz, M., and B. Metzger. 2006. Gestational diabetes mellitus. In D. C. Dale and

*D. D. Federman, eds., ACP Medicine, sec. 9, chap. 4. New York: WebMD.

*Bell, D., and J. Alele. 1997. Diabetic ketoacidosis: Why early detection and aggressive treatment are crucial. Postgraduate Medical Journal 101 (9): 193–200.

*Buchanan, T., A. Xiang, S. Kjos, and R. Watanabe. 2007. What is gestational diabe-tes? Diabetes Care 30 (Suppl. 2): S105–S111.

*Buse, J., K. Polonsky, and C. Burant. 2008. Type 2 diabetes mellitus. In P. R. Larsen et al., eds., Williams Textbook of Endocrinology, 11th ed., 1329–81. Philadelphia: Saunders Elsevier.

*Capell, P. 2004. Case study: Hemachromatosis in type 2 diabetes. Clinical Diabetes 22:101–102.

*Diabetes in Control. 2005. New type 3 diabetes discovered. Author website. diabetesincontrol.com/index.php?option=com_content&view-article&id=2582.

*De Felice, F., M. Vieira, T. Bomfim, H. Decker, P. Velasco, M. Lambert, K. Viola, W.-Q. Zhao, S. Ferreira, and W. Klein. 2009. Protection of synapses against

*Alzheimer's-linked toxins: Insulin signaling prevents the pathogenic binding of AB oligomers. Proceedings of the National Academy of Sciences 106 (18): 7678.

*Peters, A. 2005. Conquering diabetes: A complete program for prevention and treatment. New York: Plume.

*Robertson, G. L. 2003. What is diabetes insipidus? Diabetes Insipidus Foundation Inc. website. www.diabetesinsipidus.org/whatisdi.htm.

*Smeltzer, S., and B. Bare. 2004. Medical-surgical nursing. Vol. 2. 10th ed. (Philippine). Philadelphia: Lippincott.

*Steenhuysen, J. 2009. Insulin protects brain from Alzheimer's: U.S. study. UK Reuters website. http://uk.reuters.com/article/idUKN0253100820090202.

*Allen C., T. LeCaire, M. Palta, K. Daniels, M. Meredith, and D. D'Alessio. 2001. Risk factors for frequent and severe hypoglycemia in type 1 diabetes. Diabetes Care 24 (11): 1878–81.

*American Diabetes Association. 2004. Smoking and diabetes: Clinical practice recommendations 2004. Diabetes Care 27 (Suppl. 1): S74–S75.

*American Diabetes Association. 2008. The genetics of diabetes. Author website. www.diabetes.org/genetics.jsp.

*Bristow, I. R., and M. C. Spruce. 2009. Fungal foot infection, cellulitis and diabetes: A review. Diabetic Medicine 26 (5): 548–51.

*Clarke W., L. Gonder-Frederick, F. Richards, and P. Cryer. 1991. Multifactorial ori-gin of hypoglycemic symptom unawareness in

IDDM: Association with defective glucose counter-regulation and better glycemic control. Diabetes 40:680–85.222

*Cryer, P. E. 2004. Diverse causes of hypoglycemia-associated autonomic failure in diabetes. New England Journal of Medicine 350 (22): 2272–79.

*Ganda, P. 1980. Pathogenesis of macro-vascular disease in the human diabetic, Diabetes 29:931–42.

*Giovannucci, E., E. Rimm, M. Stampfer, G. Colditz, and W. Willett. 1998. Diabetes mellitus and risk of prostate cancer (United States). Cancer Causes and Control 9 (1): 3–9.

*Harjutsalo, V., S. Katoh, C. Sarti, N. Tajima, and J. Tuomilehto. 2004. Population-based assessment of familial clustering of diabetic nephropathy in Type 1 diabetes. Diabetes 53:2449–54.

*Hawkins, M., and L. Rossetti. 2005. Insulin resistance and its role in the pathogenesis of type 2 diabetes. In Joslin's Diabetes Mellitus, 14th ed., 425–48. Philadelphia: Lip-pincott.

*Jones, M., R. Drut, M. Valencia, and A. Mijalovsky. 2005. Empty sella syndrome, panhypopituitarism, and diabetes insipidus. Fetal and Pediatric Pathology 24 (3): 191–204.

*Liu, S., S. Chen, K. Chang, and J. Wang. 2004. Brain abscess presenting as postpartum diabetes insipidus. Taiwanese Journal of Obstetrics and Gynecology 43 (1): 46–49.

*Mayo Clinic staff. October 11, 2008. Diabetes symptoms: When to consult your doc-tor. Mayo-Clinic website. mayoclinic.com/health/diabetes-symptoms/DA00125.

*Medical News Today. 2006. Type 1 diabetes: Worldwide study looks to find causes. www.medicalnewstoday.com/articles/37702.php.

*Remuzzi, G., A Schieppati, and P. Ruggenenti. 2002. Clinical practice: Nephropathy in patients with type 2 diabetes. New England Journal of Medicine 346 (15): 1145–51.

*Schoenstadt, A. 2008. Symptoms of diabetes. EMedTV website. http://diabetes.emedtv.com/diabetes/symptoms-of-diabetes.html.

*Smyth, D., V. Plagnol, N. Walker, J. Cooper, K. Downes, J. Yang, J. Howson, H. Stevens, R. McManus, C. Wijmenga, G. Heap, P. Dubois, D. Clayont, J. Hunt,

*D. van Heel, and J. Todd. 2008. Shared and distinct genetic variants in type 1 diabetes and celiac disease. Pub Med website. www.ncbi.nlm.nih.gov/pubmed/19073967.

*Tabibiazar, R., and S. Edelman. 2003. Silent ischemia in people with diabetes: A condition that must be heard. Clinical Diabetes 21 (1): 5–9.

*Takasawa, H., Y. Takahashi, M. Abe, K. Osame, S. Watanabe, T. Hisatake, K. Ya-suda, Y. Kaburagi, H. Kajio, and M. Noda. 2007. An elderly case of type 2 diabetes which developed in association with oral and esophageal candidiasis. Internal Medi-cine 46 (7): 387–89.

*Tintinalli, J., D. Gabor, and J. Stapczynski. 2003. Emergency medicine: A comprehensive study guide. 6th Ed. New York: McGraw-Hill Professional.

*Willis, J. 2009. Causes of diabetes. Sclero website. www.sclero.org/medical/symptoms/associated/diabetes/causes.ht ml.

*Zochodne, D. W. 2001. Peripheral nerve disease. In H. C. Gerstein, R. B. Haynes, eds., Evidence-based diabetes care, 466–87. Hamilton, ON: B. C. Decker.

* ACUPOINT POCKET REFERENCE by Bob Flaws ISBN 0-936185-93-7.

* CHINESE MEDICINAL TEAS: Simple, Proven, Folk Formulas for Common Diseases & Promoting Healthby Zong Xiao-fan & Gary Liscum ISBN 0-936185-76-7.

* CHINESE PEDIATRIC MASSAGE THERAPY: A Parent's & Practitioner's Guide to the Prevention & Treatmentof Childhood Illness by Fan Ya-li.

* ACUPUNCTURE PHYSICAL MEDICINE: An Acupuncture Touch point Approach to the Treatment of Chronic Pain, Fatigue, and Stress Disorders by Mark Seem.

* GOLDEN NEEDLE WANG LE-TING: A 20th Century Master's Approach to Acupuncture by Yu Hui-chan & Han Fu-ru,trans. by Shuai Xue-zhong.

* THE DIVINE FARMER'S MATERIA MEDICA: A Translation of the Shen Nong Ben Caotranslation by Yang Shouz-zhong.

* THE DIVINELY RESPONDING CLASSIC: A Translation of the Shen Ying Jing from ZhenJiu Da Chengtrans. By Yang Shou-zhong & Liu Feng-ting.

* Mitka, M. 2007. Poor patient adherence may undermine aim of continuous glucose monitoring. Journal of the American Medical Association 298 (6): 614–15.

*National Diabetes Information clearing house. 2008. Diagnosis of diabetes. Author website: http://diabetes.niddk.nih.gov/dm/pubs/diagnosis/index.htm.

*Peters, A. 2005. Conquering diabetes: A complete program for prevention and treatment, New York: Plume.

*Porcellati, F. 2003. Counter regulatory hormone and symptom responses to insulin-induced hypoglycemia in the postprandial state in humans. Diabetes 52 (11): 2774–83.

*Sapountzi, P., G. Charnogursky, M. Emanuele, D. Murphy, F. Nabhan, and N.

*Emanuele. 2005. Case study: Diagnosis of insulinoma using continuous glucose monitoring system in a patient with diabetes. Clinical Diabetes 23:140–43.

*Schrot, R., K. Patel, and P. Foulis. 2007. Evaluation of inaccuracies in the measurement of glycemia in the laboratory, by glucose meters, and through measurement of hemoglobin A1C. Clinical Diabetes 25:43–49.

*Shlipak, M. 2008. Diabetic-nephropathy: Online version of BMJ Clinical Evidence. www.clinicalevidence.com.

*U.S. Preventive Services Task Force. 2008. Screening for gestational diabetes mellitus. www.ahrq.gov/clinic/uspstf/uspsgdm.htm.

* American Diabetes Association. 2006. Pancreas and islet transplantation in type 1 dia-betes: Position statement. Diabetes Care 29 (4): 935.

*American Diabetes Association. 2008. Standards of medical care in diabetes. Clinical practice recommendations: 2008. Diabetes Care 31 (Suppl. 1): S3–S110.

*Briscoe, V., and S. Davis. 2006. Hypoglycemia in type 1 and type 2 diabetes: Physiol-ogy, pathophysiology, and management. Clinical Diabetes 24:115–21.

*Cheng, A. Y. Y., and B. Zinman. 2005. Principles of insulin therapy. In Joslin's Diabetes Mellitus: 14th ed., 659–70. Philadelphia: Lippincott.

*Decker, S., C. Burt, and J. Sisk. 2009. Trends in diabetes treatment patterns among primary care providers. Journal of Ambulatory Care Management 32 (4): 333–41.

*Fowler, M. J. 2009. Inpatient diabetes management. Clinical Diabetes 27:119–22.

*Gabbe, S., and C. Graves. 2003. Management of diabetes mellitus complicating preg-nancy. Obstetrics and Gynecology 102 (4): 857–68.

*Guthrie, R. 2001. Is there a need for better basal insulin? Clinical Diabetes 19:66–70.

*Hod, M., and Y. Yogev. 2007. Goals of metabolic management of gestational diabetes. Diabetes Care 30 (Suppl. 2): S180–S187.

*Peters, A. 2005. Conquering diabetes: A complete program for prevention and treatment. New York: Plume.

*Pickup, J., and H. Keen. 2002. Continuous subcutaneous insulin infusion at 25 years. Diabetes Care 25 (30): 593–98.

*Stevens, R., S. Matsumoto, and C. Marsh. 2001. Is islet transplantation a realistic therapy for the treatment of type 1 diabetes in the near future? Clinical Diabetes 19:51–60.

*UK Prospective Diabetes Study Group. 1998. Intensive blood-glucose control with sulphonylureas or insulin compared with conventional treatment and risk of com-plications in patients with type 2 diabetes UKPDS 33: Lancet 352:461–62.

*Van Acker, K., D. De Bacquer, S. Weiss, K. Matthys, H. Raemen, C. Mathieu, and

*I. Colin. 2009. Prevalence and impact on quality of life of peripheral neuropathy with or without neuropathic pain in type 1 and type 2 diabetic patients attending hospital outpatients clinics. Diabetes and Metabolism 35 (3): 206–13.

*Vernon, M., and J. Eberstein. 2004. Atkins diabetes revolution. New York: HarperCollins.

*White, J., and R. Campbell. 2001. Recent developments in the pharmacological reduc-tion of blood glucose in patients with Type 2 diabetes. Clinical Diabetes 19:153–59.

*White, J., S. Davis, R. Cooppan, M. Davidson, K. Mulcahy, G. Manko, D. Nelinson, and the Diabetes Consortium Medical Advisory Board. 2003. Clarifying the role of insulin in type 2 diabetes management. Clinical Diabetes 21:14–21.

*White, S., R. James, S. Swift, R. Kimber, and M. Nicholson. 2001. Human islet cell transplantation: Future prospects. Diabetic Medicine 18 (2): 78–103.

References

*Dweck, C. 2006. Mindset. New York: Random House.

*Dweck, C., and P. Smiley. 1994. Individual differences in achievement goals among young children. Child Development 65 (6): 1723–43.

*Erdley, C., K. Cain, C. Loomis, F. Dumas-Hines, and C. Dweck. 2007. Relations among children's social goals, implicit personality theories, and responses to social failure. Developmental Psychology 33 (2): 263–72.

*Harris, M., D. Mertlich, and J. Rothweiler. 2001. Parenting children with diabetes. Diabetes Spectrum 14 (4): 182–84.

*Hviid, A., M. Stellfeld, J. Wohlfahrt, and M. Melbye. 2004. Childhood vaccination and type 1 diabetes. New England Journal of Medicine 350 (14): 1398–1404.

*Juvenile Diabetes Research Foundation International. 2007. Monogenic diabetes. Author website. monogenicdiabetes.org/whatis.html.

*Kamins, M., and C. Dweck. 1999. Person vs. process praise and criticism: Implications for contingent self-worth and coping. Developmental Psychology 35:835–47.

*Kirpichnikov, D., S. McFarlane, and J. Sowers. 2002. Metformin: An update. Annals of Internal Medicine 137:25.

*Levetan, C. 2001. Into the mouths of babes: The diabetes epidemic in children. Clini-cal Diabetes 19:102–4.

*Levine, B., B. Anderson, D. Butler, J. Antisdel, J. Brackett, and L. Laffel. 2001. Pre-dictors of glycemic control and short term adverse outcomes in youth with type 1 diabetes. Journal of Pediatrics 139 (2): 197–203.

*Northam, E., D. Rankins, A. Lin, R. Wellard, G. Pell, S. Finch, G. Werther, and F.

*Cameron. 2009. Central nervous system function in youth with Type 1 diabetes 12 years after disease onset. Diabetes Care 32:445–50.

*Rapaport, W. 1998. When diabetes hits home: The whole family's guide to emotional health. Alexandria, VA: American Diabetes Association.

*Renukuntla, V., K. Hassan, S. Wheat, and R. Heptulla. 2009. Disaster preparedness in pediatric type 1 diabetes mellitus. Pediatrics 124 (5): e973–77.

*Rewers, A., P. Chase, T. Mackenzie, P. Walravens, M. Roback, M. Rewers,

*R. Hamman, and G. Klingensmith. 2002. Predictors of acute complications in children with type 1 diabetes. Journal of the American Medical Association 287 (19): 2511–18.

*Rosenbloom, A., and J. Silverstein. 2003. Type 2 diabetes in children and adolescents. Alexandria, VA: American Diabetes Association.

*Rothman, R., S. Mulvaney, T. Elasy, T. Gebretsadik, A. Shintani, A. Potter, W.

*Russell, and D. Schlundt. 2008. Self-management behaviors, racial disparities, and glycemic control among adolescents with type 2 diabetes. Pediatrics 121 (4): e912–19.226   References

*Silverstein, J., G. Klingensmith, K. Copeland, L. Plotnick, F. Kaufman, L. Laffel, L.

*Deeb, M. Grey, B. Anderson, L. Holzmeister, and N. Clark. 2005. Care of children and adolescents with type 1 diabetes. Diabetes Care 28 (1): 186–212.

*Travis L., B. Brouhard, and B. Schreiner. 1987. Diabetes mellitus in children and adoles-cents. Philadelphia: W. B. Saunders.

*Vernon, M., and J. Eberstein. 2004. Atkins diabetes revolution. New York: HarperCollins.

Published by IMB Publishing 2014

CPSIA information can be obtained
at www.ICGtesting.com
Printed in the USA
BVHW092110310719

554786BV00009B/218/P